The Complete Anti-Inflammatory Cookbook For Gut Health & Immunity: 125 Nutritionist-Verified Recipes To Provide Rapid Relief & Results For Gut Health Immunity, Plus Easy-To-Follow 21-Day Meal Plan With Organic, Nutrient-Rich & Safe Ingredients For Gut Health Immunity.

EMPIRE Publishing
20212 Champion Forest Dr. #303
Spring, TX 77379
www.empireghostwriter.com/book-process
@empirepubishing

Legal & Disclaimer

TABLE OF CONTENTS

Introduction...I

CHAPTER TWO: Snacks...1
   Tangy Tomato Soup...2
   Oat And Wheat Cookies..3
   Chocolate Peanut Cookies...4
   Maple Oatmeal Bread..5
   German Dark Bread..6
   Onion And Garlic Wheat Bread...7
   White Chocolate-Cranberry Cookies..8
   Whole-Wheat–Chocolate Chip Cookies...9
   Good-For-You Chocolate Chip Cookies..10
   Oatmeal Sunflower Bread..11
   Southwest Stuffed Avocado Bowls...12
   Flaxseed Yogurt...14
   Raw Lemon Pie Bars..15
   Trail-Mix Energy Bars..16
   Zucchini Balls With Capers And Bacon...18
   Sweet Orange And Lemon Barley Risotto...20
   Homemade Applesauce...21
   Boiled Peanuts...22
   Homemade Beet Hummus..23
   Coconut Pudding With Tropical Fruit...25
   Sweet Coconut Cassava..26
   Tofu With Salted Caramel Pearls..27
   Homemade Hummus...28
   Corn Coconut Pudding..30
   Berry Jam With Chia Seeds..31
   Apple Risotto...32

CHAPTER THREE: Breakfast...33
   Gut-Healing Smoothie...34
   Aloe-Mint Smoothie..35
   Cinnamon Berry Smoothie..36
   Spinach and Aloe Smoothie..37
   Berry Flax Smoothie..38
   Strawberry Healthy Gut Smoothie...39

TABLE OF CONTENTS

Apple-Banana Smoothie...40
Turmeric Latte..41
Herb Scrambled Egg with Asparagus..................................42
Sausage and Sauerkraut..44
Banana, Flax and Turmeric Oats...45
Sweet Miso Porridge..46
Fruity Ginger Juice...47
Pear & Celery Juice..48
Apple & Cucumber Juice...49
Kiwi, Apple & Cucumber Juice...50
Broccoli, Apple & Orange Juice...51
Orange & Kale Juice...52
Pear & Fennel Juice..53
Apple, Orange & Swiss Chard Juice...................................54
Carrot, Beet & Apple Juice...55
Apple, Pear & Carrot Juice...56
Apple, Pear & Orange Juice...57
Kiwi, Apple & Grapes Juice...58
Peach & Oat Smoothie...59
Apple Oat Smoothie...60
Strawberry Oat Smoothie..61
Blackberry Smoothie..62
Blueberry & Avocado Smoothie..63
Date & Almond Smoothie..64
Pear & Almond Smoothie..65
Mango, Orange & Cucumber Smoothie.............................66
Raspberry Oat Smoothie...67
Kiwi & Oat Smoothie...68
Apple & Spinach Smoothie...69
Cucumber & Celery Smoothie...70

CHAPTER FOUR: Lunch...71
Mushroom & Beef Bone Broth..72
Shiitake-Miso Cod Soup..74
Vegetable-Coconut Curry Soup...76
Deviled Egg Salad...78
Carrot and Beet Coleslaw...79

TABLE OF CONTENTS

Hearty Winter Salad with Forbidden Rice..80
Roasted Vegetable and White Bean Salad...81
Pumpkin Seed Pesto Chicken and Arugula Sandwich.....................83
Hummus Vegetable Sandwich..85
Green Goddess Cucumber Tea Sandwiches...87
Shrimp with Beans...89
Broccoli Fritters...90
Roasted Broccoli...91
Roasted Maple Carrots...92
Sweet & Tangy Green Beans..93
Sautéed Carrots and Beans...94
Antipasto on a Stick..95
Crab and Miso Soup..96
Mexican Lime Chicken...97
Pad Thai Noodles..98
Parmesan Coated Wings... 99
Pina Colada Bites..100
Savory Chicken and Rice Muffins..101
Tuesday Tacos..102
Turkey Burgers with Spinach and Feta...103
Minestrone...104
Cheesy Chicken Fritters..106
Crispy Falafel..107
Chicken Alfredo Pasta Bake...109

CHAPTER FIVE: Dinner..111
Cheeseburger Macaroni...112
Salmon Skewers...114
Lemon Chicken...115
Dijon Chicken Thighs...116
Delicious Taco Chicken...117
Easy Broiled Fish Fillet..118
Baked Tomato Basil Fish...119
Flavorful Grilled Shrimp..120
Chicken Kababs..121
Baked Salmon...122
Baked Chicken Wings...123

TABLE OF CONTENTS

Spicy Lemon Chicken..124
Bowl With Cashew Tahini Sauce...125
Rice Bean Freezer Burritos 127
Roasted Veggie Hummus Pita Pockets...129
Sausage Peppers Baked Ziti...130
Sauteed Butternut Squash 132
Spiced Sweet Potato Wedges..133
Stetson Chopped Salad...135
Stuffed Sweet Potato With Hummus Dressing.................................137
Sweet Savory Hummus Plate..138
Sweet Potato Black Bean Chili For Two...139
Tomato Artichoke Gnocchi...141
Vegan Buddha Bowl..143
Vegan Cauliflower Fried Rice..145
Oatmeal Bread To Live For...147
Vermicelli Puttanesca...148
Spinach And Artichoke Dip Pasta..149
Grilled Eggplant..150
Tex-Mex Bean Tostadas..152

CHAPTER SIX: Desserts..153
Millet Chocolate Pudding...154
Vanilla Maple Chia Pudding...155
Dark Chocolate Gelato..156
Bread Pudding with Blueberries...157
Chocolate English Custard Recipes..158
Berry Crumb Cake...159
Peanut Butter Oatmeal Chocolate Chip Cookies..............................161
Granola Bars..163
Baked Peanut Butter Protein Bars..164
Lime Cake..165
Banana Oatmeal Chocolate Chip Cookies (Healthy!)........................167
Larabar Snack Bar...169
Kulfi Indian Ice Cream..170
Easy No-Bake Key Lime Pie Recipe...171
Lemon Cheesecake Recipe (Limoncello Cake!).................................173
Dark Chocolate with Pomegranate Seeds...175

TABLE OF CONTENTS

Chocolate Butter Honey Covered Bananas...176

Hummus with Tahini and Turmeric..177

Pineapple Orange Creamsicle...178

Easy Peach Cobbler Recipe with Bisquick..179

Healthy 5-minute Strawberry Pineapple Sherbet..181

Best Coconut Milk Ice Cream (Dairy-free!)..182

Lemon Crinkle Cookies Recipe...184

The Best No-Bake Chocolate Lasagna...186

Easiest Healthy Watermelon Smoothie Recipe...188

21-Day Meal Plan..189

Day 1:...190
  Breakfast: Gut-Healing Smoothie..34
  Snacks: Tangy Tomato   Soup...2
  Lunch: Mushroom & Beef Bone Broth..72
  Snacks: Good-For-You Chocolate Chip Cookies..10
  Dinner: Cheeseburger Macaroni...112
  Dessert: Millet Chocolate Pudding...154

Day 2:...190
  Breakfast: Aloe-Mint Smoothie..35
  Snacks: Oat And Wheat Cookies...3
  Lunch: Shiitake-Miso Cod Soup..72
  Snacks: Oatmeal Sunflower Bread..11
  Dinner: Salmon Skewers..114
  Dessert: Vanilla Maple Chia Pudding...155

Day 3:...190
  Breakfast: Cinnamon Berry Smoothie...36
  Snacks: Maple Oatmeal Bread...5
  Lunch: Vegetable-Coconut Curry Soup..76
  Snacks: Southwest Stuffed Avocado Bowls..12
  Dinner: Lemon Chicken...115
  Dessert: Dark Chocolate Gelato..156

TABLE OF CONTENTS

21-Day Meal Plan..189

Day 4:...191
Breakfast: Spinach and Aloe Smoothie...37
Snacks: German Dark Bread..6
Lunch: Deviled Egg Salad..78
Snacks: Flaxseed Yogurt...14
Dinner: Dijon Chicken Thighs..116
Dessert: Bread Pudding with Blueberries...157

Day 5:...191
Breakfast: Berry Flax Smoothie..38
Snacks: Onion And Garlic Wheat Bread...7
Lunch: Carrot and Beet Coleslaw..79
Snacks: Raw Lemon Pie Bars..15
Dinner: Delicious Taco Chicken...117
Dessert: Chocolate English Custard Recipes...158

Day 6:...191
Breakfast: Strawberry Healthy Gut Smoothie..39
Snacks: White Chocolate-Cranberry Cookies..8
Lunch: Hearty Winter Salad with Forbidden Rice.....................................80
Snacks: Trail-Mix Energy Bars..16
Dinner: Easy Broiled Fish Fillet..118
Dessert: Berry Crumb Cake..159

Day 7:...192
Breakfast: Apple-Banana Smoothie...40
Snacks: Whole-Wheat–Chocolate Chip Cookies...9
Lunch: Roasted Vegetable and White Bean Salad.....................................81
Snacks: Zucchini Balls With Capers And Bacon..18
Dinner: Baked Tomato Basil Fish...119
Dessert: Peanut Butter Oatmeal Chocolate Chip Cookies.......................161

TABLE OF CONTENTS

21-Day Meal Plan..189

Day 8:..192
Breakfast: Turmeric Latte..41
Snacks: Good-For-You Chocolate Chip Cookies............................10
Lunch: Pumpkin Seed Pesto Chicken and Arugula Sandwich.........83
Snacks: Sweet Coconut Cassava...26
Dinner: Flavorful Grilled Shrimp..120
Dessert: Granola Bars...163

Day 9:..192
Breakfast: Herb Scrambled Egg with Asparagus...............................42
Snacks: Oatmeal Sunflower Bread...11
Lunch: Hummus Vegetable Sandwich..85
Snacks: Tofu With Salted Caramel Pearls...27
Dinner: Chicken Kababs..121
Dessert: Lime Cake...165

Day 10:..193
Breakfast: Sausage and Sauerkraut...44
Snacks: Southwest Stuffed Avocado Bowls.......................................12
Lunch: Green Goddess Cucumber Tea Sandwiches...........................87
Snacks: Homemade Hummus..28
Dinner: Baked Chicken Wings..123
Dessert: Larabar Snack Bar..169

Day 11:..193
Breakfast: Banana, Flax and Turmeric Oats......................................45
Snacks: Flaxseed Yogurt...14
Lunch: Shrimp with Beans...89
Snacks: Corn Coconut Pudding...30
Dinner: Stuffed Sweet Potato With Hummus Dressing......................137
Dessert: Lemon Cheesecake Recipe (Limoncello Cake!)..................173

TABLE OF CONTENTS

21-Day Meal Plan..189

Day 12:...193
Breakfast: Sweet Miso Porridge 46
Snacks: Raw Lemon Pie Bars..15
Lunch: Broccoli Fritters...90
Snacks: Berry Jam With Chia Seeds.....................................31
Dinner: Sweet Savory Hummus Plate.................................138
Dessert: Hummus with Tahini and Turmeric.....................177

Day 13:...194
Breakfast: Hummus with Tahini and Turmeri.......................47
Snacks: Trail-Mix Energy Bars...16
Lunch: Roasted Broccoli...91
Snacks: Apple Risotto...32
Dinner: Sweet Potato Black Bean Chili For Two................139
Dessert: Pineapple Orange Creamsicle..............................178

Day 14:...194
Breakfast: Pear & Celery Juice..48
Snacks: Zucchini Balls With Capers And Bacon...................18
Lunch: Roasted Maple Carrots..92
Snacks: Tangy Tomato   2
Soup..   141
Dinner: Tomato Artichoke Gnocchi.....................................179
Dessert: Easy Peach Cobbler Recipe with Bisquick...............
                                                                                              194

Day 15:... 49
Breakfast: Apple & Cucumber Juice......................................20
Snacks: Sweet Orange And Lemon Barley Risotto...............93
Lunch: Sweet & Tangy Green Beans....................................... 3
Snacks: Oat And Wheat Cookies...143
Dinner: Vegan Buddha Bowl...181
Dessert: Healthy 5-minute Strawberry Pineapple Sherbet..........

TABLE OF CONTENTS

21-Day Meal Plan..189

Day 16:..195
Breakfast: Kiwi, Apple & Cucumber Juice..50
Snacks: Homemade Applesauce..21
Lunch: Sautéed Carrots and Beans..94
Snacks: Maple Oatmeal Bread..5
Dinner: Vegan Cauliflower Fried Rice..145
Dessert: Best Coconut Milk Ice Cream (Dairy-free!)................................182

Day 17:..195
Breakfast: Broccoli, Apple & Orange Juice..51
Snacks: Homemade Beet Hummus..23
Lunch: Antipasto on a Stick..95
Snacks: German Dark Bread..6
Dinner: Oatmeal Bread To Live For..147
Dessert: Lemon Crinkle Cookies Recipe..184

Day 18:..195
Breakfast: Orange & Kale Juice..52
Snacks: Coconut Pudding With Tropical Fruit..25
Lunch: Crab and Miso Soup..96
Snacks: Onion And Garlic Wheat Bread..7
Dinner: Vermicelli Puttanesca..148
Dessert: The Best No-Bake Chocolate Lasagna..186

Day 19:..196
Breakfast: Pear & Fennel Juice..53
Snacks: Sweet Coconut Cassava..26
Lunch: Mexican Lime Chicken..97
Snacks: White Chocolate-Cranberry Cookies..8
Dinner: Spinach And Artichoke Dip Pasta..149
Dessert: Easiest Healthy Watermelon Smoothie Recipe..188

TABLE OF CONTENTS

21-Day Meal Plan..189

Day 20:..196
    Breakfast: Apple, Orange & Swiss Chard Juice................54
    Snacks: Tofu With Salted Caramel Pearls................27
    Lunch: Pad Thai Noodles................98
    Snacks: Whole-Wheat–Chocolate Chip Cookies................9
    Dinner: Grilled Eggplant................150
    Dessert: Baked Peanut Butter Protein Bars................164

Day 21:..196
    Breakfast: Carrot, Beet & Apple Juice................55
    Snacks: Homemade Hummus................28
    Lunch: Parmesan Coated Wings................99
    Snacks: Good-For-You Chocolate Chip Cookies................10
    Dinner: Tex-Mex Bean Tostadas................152
    Dessert: Banana Oatmeal Chocolate Chip Cookies (Healthy!)................167

CONCLUSION..197

ABOUT THE AUTHOR..201

INDEX..203

CHAPTER ONE:
Introduction

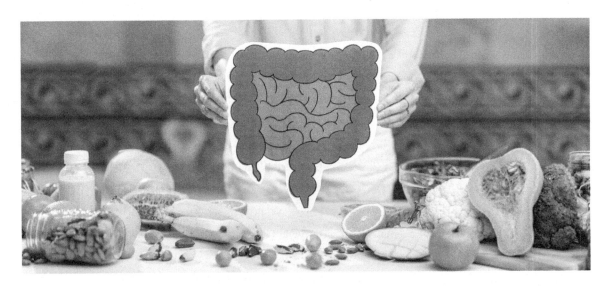

INTRODUCTION

Hippocrates said that "all disease begins in the gut," and he couldn't have been more right. Research shows that 70% of the immune system is located in the gut, where there is a veritable forest of diverse, good bacteria. Everything you eat can affect not only your weight and energy level, but also your immune system.

Cells inside of the intestinal lining excrete antibodies straight into your gut, where the bacteria inside your GI tract work to aid digestion. When a disease invades the body, the body's immune system jumps into action, and research now shows that the microbiome of bacteria and your immune system inside the gut play a big role in how your body responds to disease.

The nutrition that supports your body plays a key role in your immune system functioning. All of that nutrition and digestion starts in your gut. Immune cells interact with the microbiome in your intestinal tract and all the various bacteria that live there. The main factor that influences the diversity and healthy composition of your gut microbiome is your diet. All the bacteria in your gut helps determine the effectiveness of your immune cells.

You know that saying, "you are what you eat"? Well, that delicately balanced flora inside your gut is directly affected by the food that you put into it. Since your immune system and gut health are so vitally connected, what is inside your gut translates into how well your immune system can function.

A diverse diet can create a healthy, abundant array of bacteria inside your unique gut microbiome. Since Western diet tends to be high in animal proteins, saturated fats, sugars, and processed foods, people living in Western cultures tend to have a less diverse gut bacteria, which can lead to inflammation and chronic health conditions. So, what can you do?

Easy—you can follow the tried-and-true recipes in this cookbook to help you diversify your diet with all the right nutrients. As a result, you'll bolster your gut health and immunity.

TIME TO GUT THE DIET

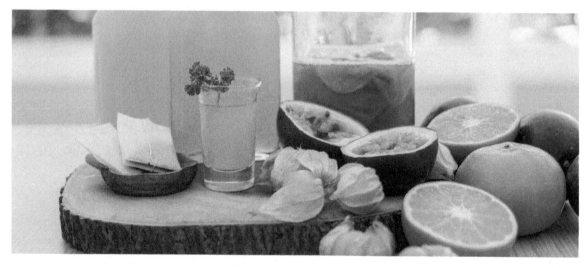

A high-fiber, plant-rich diet filled with whole grains and healthy fruits and vegetables is the framework for which to build a healthy, diverse colony of beneficial microbes. The good bacteria in your gut can help break down the fiber and stimulate immune cell activity.

The microbiome inside your gut is the vast, thick forest of literally trillions of microorganisms that live inside our bodies, with the majority being located inside the intestines. Inside the microbiome, immune activity is high, and there is a production of key antimicrobial proteins. What we eat determines what kind of microbes live inside our microbiome.

A high-fiber, plant-rich diet that includes a good variety of fruits, vegetables, and whole grains and legumes supports the functioning of the good bacteria in our gut. Furthermore, those microbes that break down the fibers into short-chain fatty acids are called prebiotics because they actually feed the microbes living within us. That's why you have probably heard how beneficial prebiotics and probiotics are for you because they contain helpful live bacteria and fibers that feed and support the tiny world of good bacteria populating your gut.

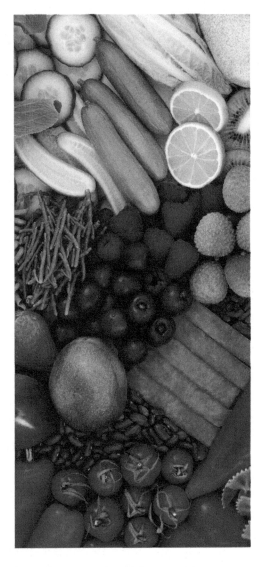

All those little bacteria play important roles in keeping you healthy and immune to outside bad bacteria and diseases that might invade your body. They metabolize the food you eat, keep your digestive system working as it should, and provide an immune barrier against intruding illnesses.

Since gut bacteria thrives on the complex carbs and fibers that it helps digest, a fiber-rich diet supports the microbiome and reduces inflammatory response.

But how do we know when we are getting enough of the nutrients we need and which ones are better than others? That's where this book comes in. Remember when you were a kid and those television ads told you to "eat a rainbow" by encouraging you to choose colors from the various food groups. Add a red apple, a splash of green broccoli, and maybe a dark brown slice of whole grain bread—toss in some orange sweet potatoes and maybe even a few dark blueberries, and you'd have an impressive variety of colors.

Well, that advice wasn't just to make your plate pretty; it's good guidance to follow! Several servings of colorful fruits and vegetables a day can also fortify the benefits of plant-based eating. Just think of how many colorful foods are also packed with fiber—from yams to apples to broccoli and beyond!

Dietary diversity promotes microbial diversity. So, the best way to make sure that your forest of good microbes is as diverse as possible is to eat a wide variety of foods. The more colorful your plate is to the eye; the better off your healthy and nutritional diet. With that in mind, let's break it down even further.

DECONSTRUCTED DISHES

A varied diet is nothing new as far as solid health advice. However, it is even more important when talking about gut health and immune cell functioning.

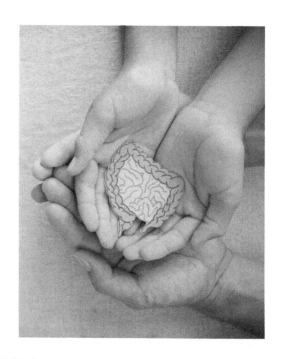

And although there isn't one "miracle food" that can ensure protection for your health, there is evidence that consistent healthy patterns and nutrient combinations in your diet can better protect your body against excess inflammation and attacks by invading bacteria.

Some nutrients such as vitamin C, D, zinc, selenium, and iron are critical for well-functioning immune cells. Protein plays a big role as well. Thankfully, these nutrients are not hard to find, as they make up plentiful plant and animal foods. And if you're vegan, don't fret! The market is filled with so many comparable alternatives that can still provide you with the essential nutrients that you need for a healthy, well-functioning immune system.

On the contrary, when you limit your diet by consuming high levels of processed foods, you can negatively affect your immune system and disturb those good intestinal microorganisms. That can result in a whole host of health problems, ranging from inflammatory responses in the gut, chronic health conditions, and weak or suppressed immunity. A deficiency of nutrients can also change the body's immune response and lead people with poor nutrition to be at a greater risk of bacterial and viral infections and diseases.

It's one thing to say that eating colorful fruits and veggies, plenty of protein, and healthy fats—all garnished with natural spices and herbs—can support great gut diversity. But before we bite off more than we can chew, we need to deconstruct this larger diet into simpler pieces we can implement on a daily basis. Let's take them one at a time.

Probiotics and prebiotics are the stars of the show when it comes to gut health. Probiotic foods contain live microorganisms that can improve and maintain the good bacteria in your gut, thereby keeping your intestinal flora in balance.

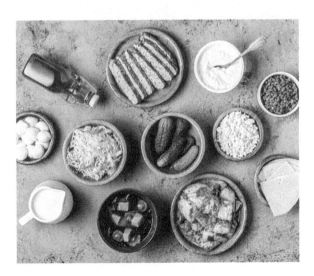

Prebiotics foods are the high-fiber foods that can feed all those hungry microflorae inside your gut.

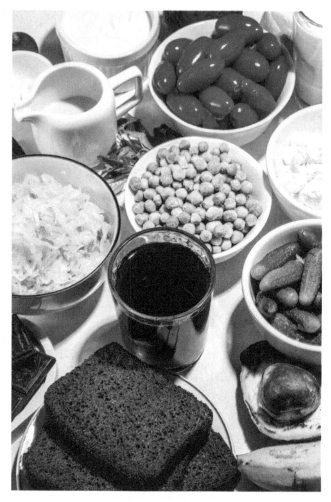

Probiotics are highly important to a top-functioning gut as they can act as an extra barrier of protection against harmful bacteria that seek to throw off your gut's natural balance. You can find probiotics in kefir, yogurt with live active cultures, and fermented foods like kimchi, sauerkraut, kombucha, and miso. All of these foods contain good probiotics that can stimulate your immune system to fight off diseases.

Prebiotic foods can include garlic, onions, asparagus, Jerusalem artichokes, dandelion greens, and bananas. Eating a wide variety of fruits and vegetables can help cover the gamut of prebiotics within a healthy diet.

Some nutrients work as antioxidants that help protect the healthy cells in your body and support the growth and activity of your immune cells. They can also aid in the production of antibodies. Vitamin C is a well-known antioxidant, and it's easy to find in citrus fruits and greens.

Some foods like grapefruits, oranges, broccoli, and kale are high in vitamin C and may increase white blood cell production, which aids in fighting off infections. Another anti-inflammatory vitamin is beta-carotene, which converts into Vitamin A and can help your body effectively respond to toxins. You can find ample amounts of this nutrient in sweet potatoes, squash, carrots, spinach, and kale.

Vitamin E can help regulate your immune system and is found in nuts, seeds, and avocado. Spinach is a superstar because not only does it have a healthy dose of Vitamin E, but it also contains Vitamin C and beta-carotene. It's what we might call a "superfood" because it has so many beneficial nutrients and properties.

Vitamin D also helps regulate immune function, and can be found in salmon, canned tuna, egg yolks, and sunshine. Too bad you can't just pour yourself a full cup of sunshine to have with breakfast each morning! Your immune cells also need zinc, a mineral that our bodies cannot produce on their own. One of the highest concentrations of zinc is found in oysters, but for those who can't stomach the thought of slurping on a half-shell, zinc is also found in shellfish, poultry, red meat, and beans.

Many foods are fortified with zinc, but it really is best to get your nutrients from raw food sources whenever possible. While you're thinking about eating fish, wild-caught fish are much healthier than the farmed varieties and pack a punch of nutrient-dense benefits.

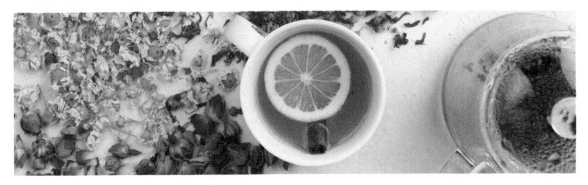

Herbal antioxidants are also important to mention. Echinacea has been shown to help boost the immune system by shortening the duration of colds and attacking some viruses like the flu. Green tea is also filled with antioxidants and amino acids that can help reduce inflammation and fight infection. If you're not a fan of plain green tea, you can still reap green tea's benefits in a naturally sweetened matcha drink.

And who could forget about garlic? Garlic has long been touted as having strong antiviral and antimicrobial properties. Garlic is another superpowered nutrient because it not only helps stimulate the immune cells into fighting disease, but it can also boost the production of T-cells and reduce stress hormones. Stress can suppress your immune system and keep it from working properly.

Using natural herbs and spices to flavor your foods is a great way to support gut diversity, as is adding healthy fats to support immune function. Olive, avocado, and canola oils can add flavor and immune-boosting benefits, so it's a win-win!

A healthy immune system also relies heavily on getting enough protein. The muscles in your body rely on protein. Since muscle consists of protein, it's important to make sure that you're getting enough protein in your diet.

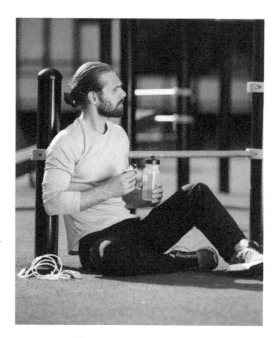

Some obvious sources of protein come from animal products, but there is good news for those of us who are vegans: plant sources are actually a better source of protein when it comes to your gut microbiome! Some research points to the benefit of eating protein with every meal.

And we can't forget about another essential food—water!

Water helps the lymphatic system and carries white blood cells throughout the body. Furthermore, you don't just have to drink water in order to get enough water into your diet, which is good news for people who struggle meeting their daily water goals. Certain foods like cucumbers, watermelon, and celery have a high water composition.

If you struggle with drinking enough water, you can also try adding a splash of lemon or infuse your water with mint or coconut, thus creating an even more beneficial drink with multiple health-boosting properties. Proper hydration is essential for getting all those important nutrients flowing to the cells they need to reach all throughout your body.

ONE SIZE DOES NOT FIT ALL

This cookbook is a grimoire of sorts—compiling all the best recipes for a wide variety of delicious, immune-boosting, gut-supporting dishes. Here, we've gathered an impressive assortment of interesting foods. And since you are your own person with your individual tastes and needs, we've made this cookbook a comprehensively curated collection of innovative ideas.

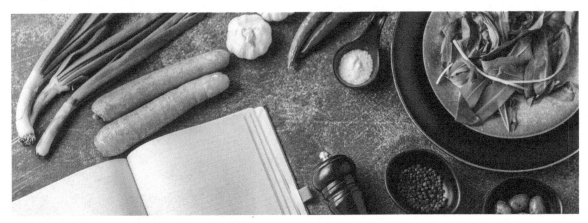

That being said, we want to touch on the premise of the Mediterranean-style diet, as the "bones" of this diet are suggested to help all that good bacteria in your gut thrive. The Mediterranean-style diet is rich in plant-based foods, fruits, vegetables, grains, legumes, fish, and nuts. It has been found in some research to decrease inflammation and support a healthy microbiome in your gut.

As with other research, plant-based diets have been linked to protecting against intestinal diseases. The main components of this style of diet can help break down and synthesize essential nutrients while reducing intestinal inflammation.

It's no secret that a diet rich in red meats, refined sugars, and fattening foods can lead to higher inflammation and hurt the bacteria colony in your gut. This diet can also increase your risk of disease, whereas plant-based diets that support the immune system can benefit the digestive system, which, in turn, may lead to increased longevity. Altogether, a healthy intestinal system and a flourishing microbiome of good bacteria in your gut may help ward off many chronic and potentially life-threatening diseases.

And although there is no single food nor single diet that can protect you against illness and supercharge your immune system, there are certainly smart steps you can take to ensure that you are feeding your body with the nutrients that will keep you healthy for many, many years to come. And speaking of tools— you're holding a great one in your hands right now!

TIME TO GET TO WORK

Work? We can already see you cringing from the other side of this book! We know you don't want more on your plate that you have to research, prepare, and put into action. You already have some great tools—information about what kinds of foods to eat to support a healthy gut immune and this cookbook to help guide you ever step of the way!

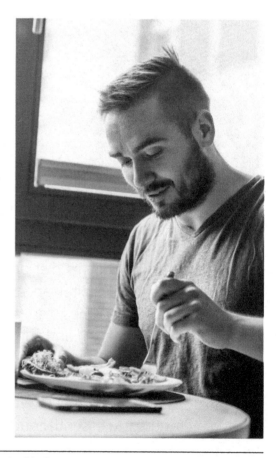

Your only job is to practice some mindful eating, relax, and derive pleasure from your food, reaping the benefits that decreased stress will have on your immune. You don't need to put in the work here because we have already done it for you.

The Complete Anti-Inflammatory Cookbook For Gut Health & Immunity

Not only are all the recipes in this book created with the right ingredients in mind to support a healthy gut, but they have all been tried, tested, and put together in a way that makes them easily modifiable for your needs and tastes.

Every dish in this cookbook has been meticulously crafted to be delicious and innovative, and to provide as much variety in your diet as we could possibly squeeze into each and every recipe. We don't want you to have long and tedious meal prep or burdensome trips to the store to hunt down hard-to-find ingredients.

That's why we've made these dishes simple to make with easily accessible ingredients, along with a whole lot of fun and creativity to please your palate. Trust us, there isn't a single dish in this book that will bore you. We've incorporated all the tips and tricks to make your meal planning easier and to execute each dish effortlessly. We think you'll find our presentations a sight for sore eyes, and your taste buds will be jumping for joy.

Having a healthy diet that can support your body's immunity should be flavorful, tasty, and maintainable. After all, what good is a healthy diet if you find yourself not wanting to keep up with your dietary choices?

So to make your nutritional choices a consistent pattern that will help your gut's immune system regularly function at its best, the food you eat needs to be mouth-watering enough for you to want to keep eating it!

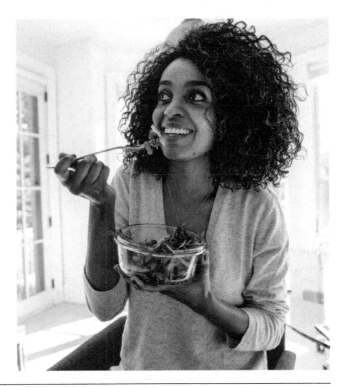

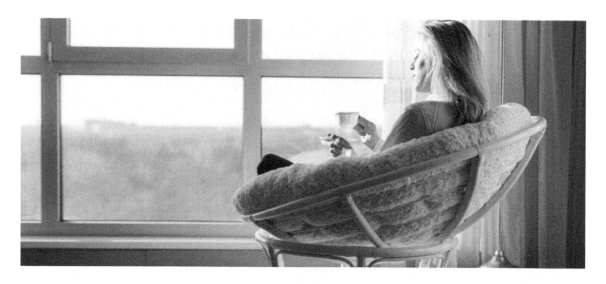

Remember, the goal here is to have a healthy, flourishing gut microbiome—a whole little world of flora inside your body that is constantly working to keep you at optimal health and fight off any invading bacteria. Therefore, you need to give your digestive system all the immune-supporting nutrients it can use to sustain itself. You and your gut are in this together, and while you are enjoying the delectable dishes in this book, your gut will be enjoying a delicately balanced biome designed to help you live your best life to the fullest for a long time to come.

Now that you have this cookbook, pour yourself a tall glass of green tea (don't forget that squeeze of lemon juice!), sit back, and flip through these pages. Pick out some appetizing and appealing recipes to get you started. Enjoy the process and savor the flavors in these recipes, while knowing that you are quite literally feeding your gut toward better health.

And when you find yourself feeling more satisfied, energized, and healthier than you've ever been, you'll know that behind every tasty bite of this cookbook are powerhouses of antioxidants and nutrients. Those bad bacteria better watch out, because you're now armed with an arsenal of recipes that will stop them in their tracks. Cheers to your stronger-than-ever immune system!

THE COMPLETE ANTI-INFLAMMATORY COOKBOOK FOR GUT HEALTH & IMMUNITY

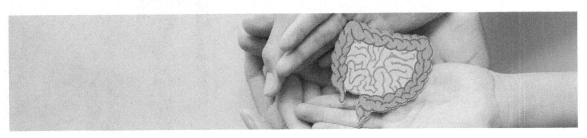

You may have heard that what goes in your mouth can affect your gut health. And although the science of these connections is still emerging, research is pointing to a close connection between those two aspects of our body. Gut bacteria is affected by what we eat, it can affect our mood, and it plays an important role in our overall health.

What is the gut microbiota?

You have trillions of bacteria in your gastrointestinal tract that make up your gut microbiota or 'the microbiome'. Your gut microbiota work together with your body to help you do a number of really important things including: breaking down and using the nutrients from food;. helping you to maintain a healthy weight; protecting your body against harmful microbes such as C. difficile and other bacteria such as E. coli; and 4) helping you to clear, absorb and fight off toxins.

These beneficial bacteria in your gut help to reduce inflammation in the gut. Inflammation is your body's natural response to injury or infection, but it can also be triggered by some foods, chemicals and infections. For example, when you use antibiotics the good gut bacteria can become depleted in some people who are able to eat a rich diet of foods that are high in prebiotics. This can lead to unhealthy inflammation of the digestive tract even though there is no infection.

There is also evidence that there is a link between the way you feed your gut bacteria and your mood. The role of the gastrointestinal tract in our emotions is referred to as the enteric nervous system. A healthy gut is also the basic foundation of a healthy body. It's no wonder that so many people feel better after they take care of their gut health.

But just like your regular health, you can only improve it by taking an active role in your lifestyle. It's not like you can stroll up to the doctor, tell them you want better gut health, and expect to leave the office with a bottle of pills.

So how can you work to improve your gut health? What can you do to make sure that your body is giving you all it has? There are various simple steps that we can take to achieve optimal gut health! Let's go over them now.

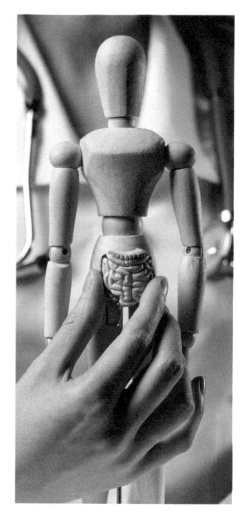

1. Drink enough water

How much water should you drink? You should drink 1-2 liters of good water a day. That's right, I said liters.

If you can't even imagine pouring that much liquid in your body, there are other ways to make sure that you get the liquid volume that is needed. Green tea is also an excellent way to hydrate your body since it contains antioxidants and nutrients. Incorporating green tea in your daily life is a much better option than drinking water since it gives you all the health benefits without the hassle.

2. Eat fermented foods

The fermentation process helps to preserve the food and kill any bacteria that could cause dangerous infections or diseases. If you're not familiar with fermented foods, they are vegetables that have been preserved through the fermentation process. Some examples of the fermented foods are sauerkraut, kimchi, and pickles!

If you enjoy eating ramen noodles then you might want to find a way to incorporate some kimchi into your soup! It's also easy to make kimchi at home by following these instructions . Now that you're familiar with fermented foods, you should be able to start incorporating them into your diet!

3. Avoid artificial sweeteners

Artificial sweeteners have been known to increase your risk of developing diabetes and obesity. These sweeteners are chemicals that are made without the use of sugar in order to decrease the calories.

They have many names like aspartame and sucralose, but they all work by tricking your body into thinking that it is getting sugar. The problem is that this causes a rise in blood sugar which can lead to some serious health problems. If your goal is better gut health then you will want to avoid these artificial sweeteners at all costs!

4. Eat a plant-based diet

If you're eating meat, eggs, dairy, and fish then you will want to make sure that you are eating a plant-based diet. The best way to observe it is that you are taking the animal out of the food, and putting plants inside instead.

This obviously promotes better gut health because your body has never been exposed to any of these foods!

5. Take probiotics regularly

Probiotics are essential to your good gut health. At first, they were only meant to be used after an infection in order to help your body fight against the illness, but these days people are taking them on a daily basis in order to increase their overall good gut health.

Here's how it works: probiotics work by countering the bad bacteria that is already inside of you and replacing it with good bacteria. If you are serious about starting a healthy gut then you should invest in a daily probiotic that is made specifically for you.

6. Eat more fiber!

Fiber is a type of carbohydrate that helps in digestion by adding bulk and moving food through your colon faster.

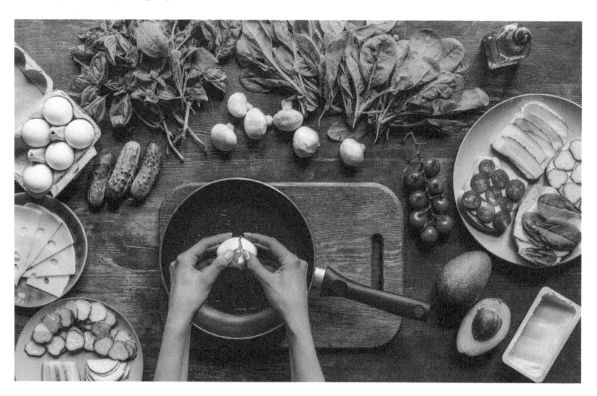

CHAPTER TWO:
Snacks

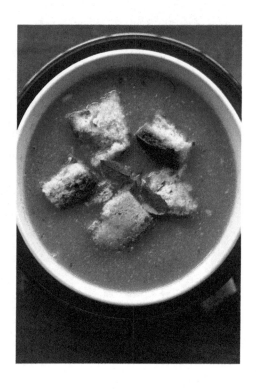

TANGY TOMATO SOUP

Preparation Time: 5 minutes
Cooking time: 30 minutes
Servings: 4

Ingredients:
- 1 large sweet onion, coarsely chopped
- 1 (28-ounce) can diced tomatoes
- 1 (28-ounce) can crushed tomatoes
- 1 cup Vegetable Broth
- 2 teaspoons dried tarragon
- 1 Medjool date, pitted and chopped (optional)
- ¼ cup balsamic vinegar

Directions:
1. Dry cook the onion over moderate to high heat with frequent turning in a big pot until it is just beginning to brown, which should take 8 to 10 minutes. Bring the tomatoes, both diced and crushed, the broth, and the tarragon to a boil after adding them.
2. Turn the heat down to low-moderate and let the mixture boil for twenty mins whereas mixing it recurrently.
3. After adding the date, purée the soup until it is completely smooth either by using an immersion blender to do so directly in the pan or by transferring the soup to a standing blender, doing so carefully, and then returning the soup to the pan.
4. After swiftly stirring the mixture, pour in the vinegar, and serve it hot.

Nutrition: *Calories 153; Fat 0g; Carbs 35g; Fiber 9g; Protein 6g*

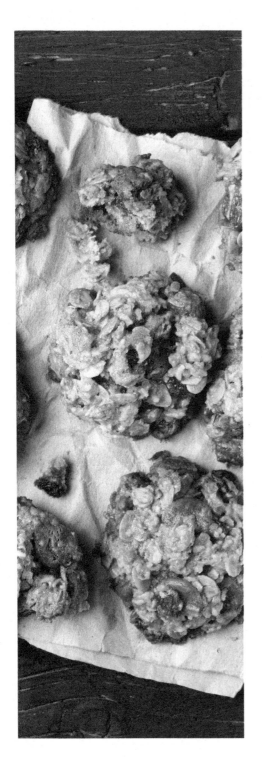

OAT AND WHEAT COOKIES

Preparation Time: 10 minutes
Cooking time: 12-15 minutes
Servings: 4

Ingredients:

- 3/4 cup (165 g) unsalted butter
- 1/2 cup (130 g) peanut butter
- 1 cup (150 g) brown sugar
- 1 ¼ cup (150 g) whole-wheat pastry flour
- 1 teaspoon baking soda
- 1 ¼ cup (100 g) rolled oats

Directions:

1. Mix all ingredients.
2. Set by rounded teaspoons onto an ungreased baking sheet.
3. Bake at 375°F (190°C, gas mark 5) for 10-12 minutes or until golden brown.
4. Let rest on the baking sheet for 1 minute and then cool on racks.

Nutrition: *Calories: 865 ; Fat: 52g; Carbs: 88g; Fiber: 9g; Protein: 15.9g*

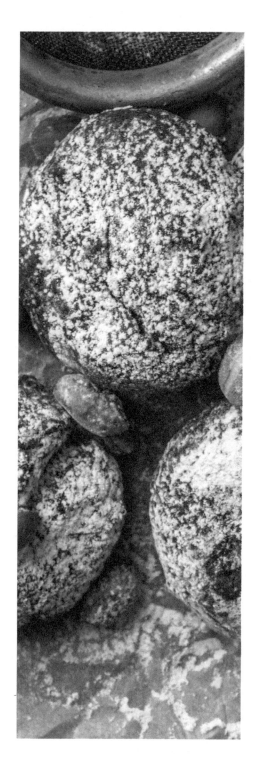

CHOCOLATE PEANUT COOKIES

Preparation Time: 10 minutes
Cooking time: 2-3 minutes
Servings: 6

Ingredients:

- 1 ounce (45 g) chocolate candy bar
- 4 tablespoons (64 g) crunchy peanut butter
- 1 cup (60 g) lightly sweetened bran cereal, such as Fiber: One

Directions:

1. Check the consistency every 30 seconds when melting the chocolate bar and the peanut butter in the oven till it is completely smooth. Take precautions to avoid getting burned.
2. Set to mix the melted chocolate and peanut butter.
3. Add cereal and gently toss until coated.
4. Drop on waxed paper or foil, making 6 cookies. Freeze for 30 minutes.
5. Put in resealable plastic bags and refrigerate.

Nutrition: *Calories: 193 ; Fat: 6g; Carbs: 25g; Fiber: 7g; Protein: 10g*

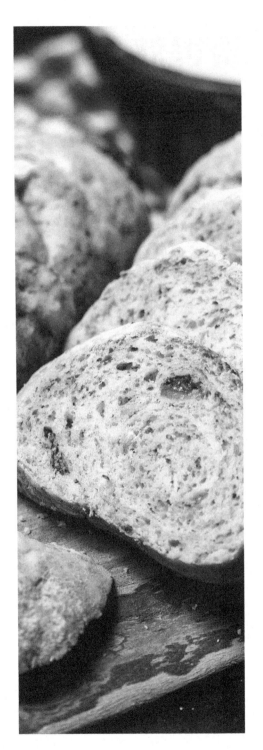

MAPLE OATMEAL BREAD

Preparation Time: 10 minutes
Cooking time: 20 minutes
Servings: 12

Ingredients:

- 1 ¾ teaspoon yeast
- 1 cup (157 ml) warm water
- 2 ½ cups (342 g) bread flour
- 1/2 cup flour
- 1 cup (27 g) rolled oats
- 1 cup (80 ml) maple syrup
- 1/4 cup (17 g) non-fat dry milk
- 2 tbsp (28 g) unsalted butter, room temperature

Directions:

1. Put all of the ingredients into the bread maker in the direction that is suggested by the creator of the bread machine.
2. Run the dough through the cycle for sweet bread or whole-wheat flour.

Nutrition: *Calories: 238; Fat: 3g; Carbs: 27g; Fiber: 6g; Protein: 21g*

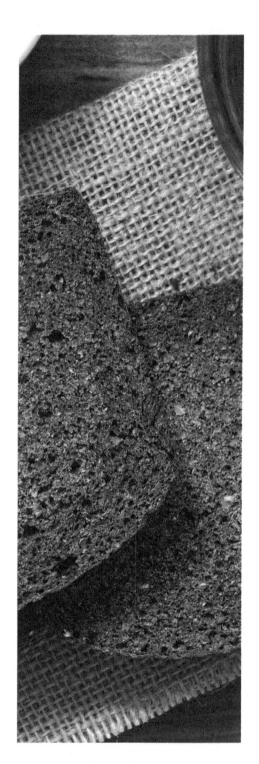

GERMAN DARK BREAD

Preparation Time: 10 minutes
Cooking time: 20 minutes
Servings: 12

Ingredients:

- 1 cup (235 ml) water
- 1/4 cup (85 g) molasses
- 1 tablespoon unsalted butter
- 2 cups (274 g) bread flour
- 1 ¼ cup (160 g) rye flour
- 2 tablespoons cocoa powder
- 1 ½ teaspoon yeast
- 1 tablespoon vital wheat gluten

Directions:

1. Put every one of the components, such as the yeast, into the bread machine in the order that was specified by the manufacturer of the bread maker. The processing should be done using a cycle designed for whole wheat.

Nutrition: *Calories: 287 ; Fat: 19g; Carbs: 18g; Fiber: 6g; Protein: 16g*

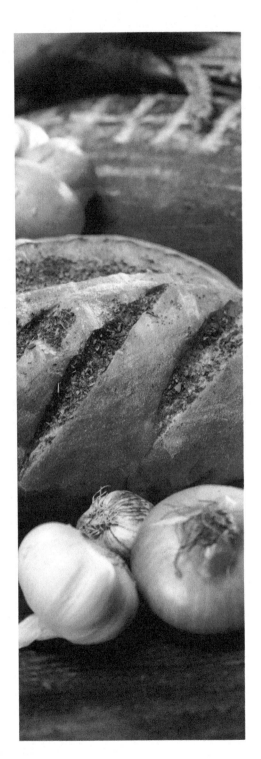

ONION AND GARLIC WHEAT BREAD

Preparation Time: 10 minutes
Cooking time: 20 minutes
Servings: 12

Ingredients:
- 1/2 cup (80 g) finely chopped onion
- 1/2 teaspoon finely chopped garlic
- 1 tablespoon sugar
- 1/2 cup whole-wheat flour
- 2 ½ cups (342 g) bread flour
- 1 ½ tablespoon non-fat dry milk
- 1 ½ teaspoon yeast
- 3/4 cup (175 ml) water
- 1 ½ tablespoon (21 g) unsalted butter

Directions:
1. Set all ingredients in the bread machine. Process on a white bread cycle.

Nutrition: *Calories: 329 ; Fat: 17g; Carbs: 9g; Fiber: 5g; Protein: 37g*

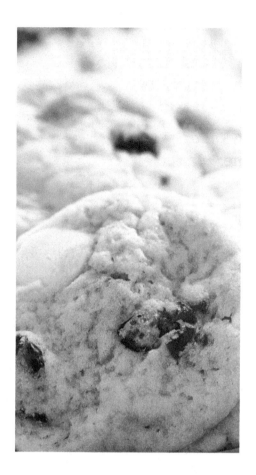

WHITE CHOCOLATE-CRANBERRY COOKIES

Preparation Time: 10 minutes
Cooking time: 10 minutes
Servings: 36

Ingredients:

- 1/2 cup (112 g) shortening
- 1 cup (225 g) brown sugar
- 1 egg
- 1 teaspoon vanilla extract
- 13/4 cups (210 g) whole-wheat pastry flour
- 1 teaspoon baking soda
- 1/4 cup (60 ml) buttermilk
- 1/2 cup (87 g) white chocolate chips
- 1/2 cup (60 g) dried cranberries

Directions:

1. Beat the shortening until light. Add sugar and beat until fluffy.
2. Mix in the egg, then stir in the vanilla.
3. Mix the items that are dry. Buttermilk should be added to them in stages as you attach them to the mixture.
4. Mix until there are no lumps. Mix in the chips as well as the cranberries.
5. Place them on a baking pane that has been spewed with non-stick vegetable oil spray and leaves approximately 2 inches (5 cm) between each one.
6. Bake for 8 to 10 minutes at 375 degrees Fahrenheit (190 degrees Celsius, or mark 5) until the top is gently browned.

Nutrition: *Calories: 361 ; Fat: 10g; Carbs: 4g; Fiber: 14g; Protein: 12g*

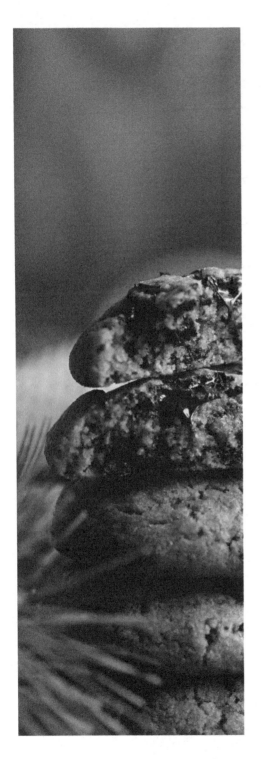

WHOLE-WHEAT–CHOCOLATE CHIP COOKIES

Preparation Time: 10 minutes
Cooking time: 10 minutes
Servings: 48

Ingredients:

- 1 cup (225 g) unsalted butter
- 1/4 cup (64 g) peanut butter
- 1 cup (340 g) honey
- 2 eggs
- 1 ½ cup whole-wheat pastry flour
- 1 teaspoon baking soda
- 2 cups (160 g) rolled oats
- 2 cups (350 g) chocolate chips
- 1 cup (110 g) chopped pecans

Directions:

1. Cream together the first 4 ingredients.
2. Add the next 5 ingredients and mix well.
3. Add enough flour for a stiff dough.
4. Drop by teaspoons on a baking sheet.
5. Bake at 375°F (190°C, gas mark 5) for 10 minutes.

Nutrition: *Calories: 365; Fat: 7g; Carbs: 67g; Fiber: 18g; Protein: 14g*

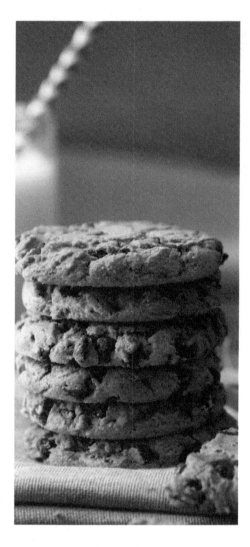

GOOD-FOR-YOU CHOCOLATE CHIP COOKIES

Preparation Time: 10 minutes
Cooking time: 10 minutes
Servings: 36

Ingredients:

- 1/4 cup (55 g) unsalted butter
- 1 cup (150 g) packed brown sugar
- 1/4 cup (85 g) honey
- 1 egg
- 1 teaspoon vanilla extract
- 1/4 cup (60 ml) skim milk
- 1 teaspoon baking soda
- 1/2 teaspoon baking powder
- 1 cup (82 g) granola
- 3/4 cup quick-cooking oats
- 2 cups whole-wheat pastry flour
- 1 cup (175 g) chocolate chips

Directions:

1. Cream the butter and brown sugar.
2. Mix in honey, egg, vanilla, milk, and baking soda and baking powder.
3. Add granola, oats, and flour. Mix all ingredients.
4. Stir in chocolate chips.
5. Place on a non-stick baking sheet in teaspoons.
6. Bake at 325°F (170°C, gas mark 3) for 10 minutes.

Nutrition: *Calories: 287; Fat: 19g; Carbs: 18g; Fiber: 6g; Protein: 3g*

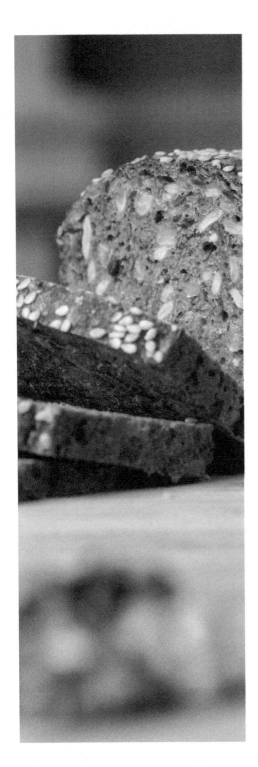

OATMEAL SUNFLOWER BREAD

Preparation Time: 10 minutes
Cooking time: 20 minutes
Servings: 12

Ingredients:
- 1 cup (235 ml) water
- 1/4 cup (85 g) honey
- 2 tablespoons (28 g) unsalted butter
- 3 cups (411 g) bread flour
- 1/2 cup (40 g) quick-cooking oats
- 2 tablespoons non-fat dry milk powder
- 2 teaspoons yeast
- 1 tablespoon vital wheat gluten
- 1/2 cup (72 g) unsalted shelled sunflower seeds

Directions:
1. In a bread machine, place entire of the components, excluding the sunflower seeds, in the order that is specified by the maker. Perform the processing using the large white loaf setting.
2. When you hear the beep, or about 5 mins before the shiatzu is finished, add the sunflower seeds.

Nutrition: *Calories: 599; Fat: 19g, Carbs: 9g, Fiber: 2g, Protein: 97g*

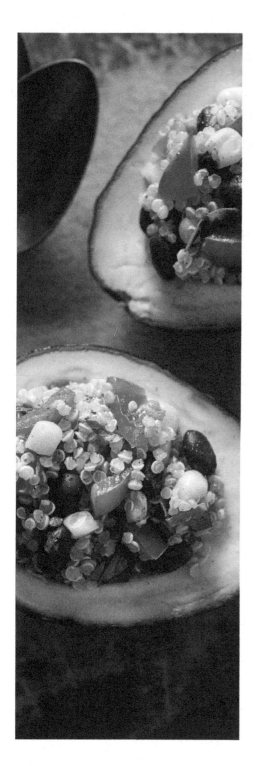

SOUTHWEST STUFFED AVOCADO BOWLS

Preparation Time: 30 minutes
Cooking time: 0 minutes
Servings: 4

Ingredients:

- 3 cups black beans (canned or cooked)
- ¾ cup chickpeas (canned or cooked)
- 1 cup water or vegetable broth (see recipe)
- ½ purple onion (chopped)
- 1 tsp. garlic powder
- ½ tsp. chili powder
- ½ tsp. cumin
- ¼ tsp. paprika
- 4 small-to-medium avocados (halved)
- 1 tsp. lime juice
- 1 pinch of salt
- ¼ cup salsa (see recipe)
- ¼ cup hummus (see recipe)

Directions:

1. When using dry beans, prepare 1 cup of dry black beans according to the method.
2. When using dry chickpeas, prepare ¼ cup of chickpeas according to the method.
3. Heat the water or vegetable broth in a medium-sized pot over medium-high heat.
4. Add the cooked black beans, chickpeas, onions, and all the spices.
5. After thoroughly combining all of the ingredients by stirring them together, boil the mixture over little temperature till almost entire water has evaporated, which should take around ten to fifteen minutes.
6. Meanwhile, sprinkle the avocado halves with lime juice and some salt.
7. Store the ingredients separately, or, serve the avocado halves with a scoop of the beans mixture and top with some hummus and salsa.

Nutrition: *Calories: 351; Fat: 20g; Carbs: 32.6g; Fiber: 15.6g; Protein: 10g*

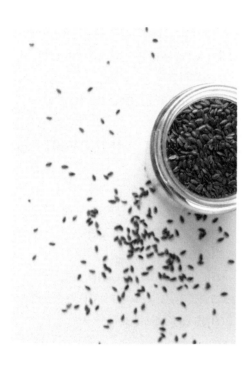

FLAXSEED YOGURT

Preparation Time: 5 minutes
Cooking time: 0 minutes
Servings: 4

Ingredients:
- 2 cups water
- ½ cup hemp seeds
- ½ cup flax seeds
- 1 cup almond milk
- 2 tsp. psyllium husk
- ¼ cup lemon juice
- ¼ tsp. stevia

Directions:
1. Soak the flax seeds. Drain the excess water.
2. Add 1 cup of boiling water to a heat-resistant blender.
3. Continue to add the dry and soaked seeds.
4. Blend the ingredients for about 4 minutes.
5. Place one more cup of water, the almond milk, and the psyllium husk in the blender and process until smooth. Remix the ingredients for another thirty seconds.
6. At long last, stir in some fresh lemon juice and stevia. Continue blending for a few more seconds.
7. Pour the flaxseed yogurt into a container and put it in the fridge.
8. Serve the flaxseed yogurt chilled and enjoy or divide the yogurt for storing.

Nutrition: *Calories: 220; Fat: 16.9g; Carbs: 9.2g; Fiber: 7.4g; Protein: 10g*

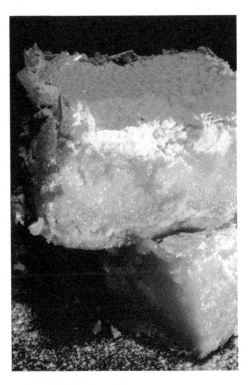

RAW LEMON PIE BARS

Preparation Time: 10 minutes
Cooking time: 0 minutes
Servings: 6

Ingredients:
- ¼ cup chia seeds
- ¼ cup pecan pieces
- ⅓ cup raw cashews
- ⅓ cup sunflower seeds
- 2 cups of pitted dates
- ½ cup vegan protein powder (vanilla flavor)
- 2 tbsp. organic lemon juice (or lime juice)
- ¼ tsp. salt

Directions:
1. Soak the chia seeds according to the method and drain the excess water.
2. Place the pecans, cashews, chia seeds, and sunflower seeds in the container of a food processor. Using the processor's blade attachment, pulse the ingredients on the lowest setting until the mixture becomes crumbly.
3. Put the dates, the juice of one lemon or lime, and some salt into a food processor. Blend until smooth. Continue to pulse the mixture while adding the protein powder until it reaches a consistency that is somewhere between chunky and doughy.
4. After transferring the dough to a baking sheet that has been covered with a piece of parchment paper, proceed to form the dough into a square with a thickness of an inch and a half by using your fingers or a rolling pin to flatten it out.
5. Place the sheet pan in the freezer and let it stay there for about an hour, until either the chunk is frozen to a solid state, whichever comes first.

Nutrition: *Calories: 272; Fat: 10.7g; Carbs: 34.9 g; Fiber: 6.5 g; Protein: 8.9 g*

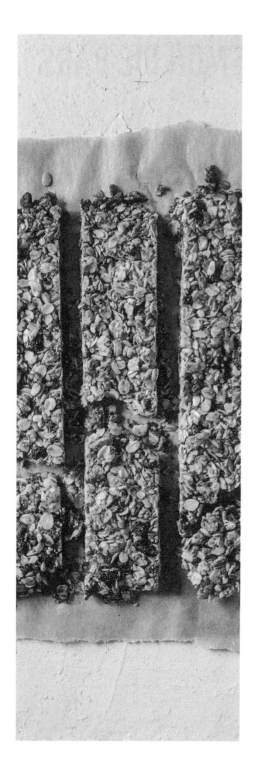

TRAIL-MIX ENERGY BARS

Preparation Time: 25 minutes
Cooking time: 0 minutes
Servings: 12

Ingredients:

- 2 cups rolled oats
- 2 cups puffed brown rice (see recipe)
- 1 cup almonds (unsalted, chopped)
- ¼ cup roasted pumpkin seeds (unsalted)
- ¼ cup hemp seeds
- Pinch of salt
- 2 cups dates (pitted)
- ½ cup agave nectar (or maple syrup)
- ¼ cup sweet cashew cheese spread (see recipe)
- 1 tbsp. vanilla extract

Directions:

1. Combine the oats, puffed rice, almonds, seeds, and salt in a large bowl.
2. Blend the dates in a food processor and pulse until finely chopped.
3. Add the chopped dates to the dry ingredients and stir.
4. Take a small saucepan and put it on low heat.
5. Combine the agave nectar and cashew cheese spread in the pan. Prevent cooking it.
6. Use a mixer to combine the heated agave and cashew mixture with the dry ingredients.
7. Mix until smooth and creamy while adding the vanilla extract.
8. Line a bread form with parchment paper and pour the mixture down into this form.
9. Store the mix in the fridge for about 1 hour, until the batter has become hard.
10. Separate the chunk into 12 or 24 bars.
11. Enjoy or store wrapped in wrapping foil.

Nutrition: *Calories: 302; Fat: 10.4g; Carbs: 44.9g; Fiber: 4.9g; Protein: 7.2g*

ZUCCHINI BALLS WITH CAPERS AND BACON

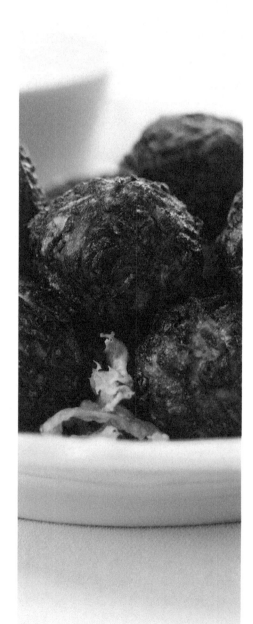

Preparation Time: 3 hours
Cooking time: 20 minutes
Servings: 10

Ingredients:

- 2 zucchinis, shredded
- 2 bacon slices, chopped
- 1/2 cup cream cheese, at room temperature
- 1 cup fontina cheese
- 1/4 cup capers
- 1 clove garlic, crushed
- 1/2 cup grated Parmesan cheese
- 1/2 tsp. poppy seeds
- 1/4 tsp. dried dill weed
- 1/2 tsp. onion powder
- Salt and black pepper, to taste
- 1 cup crushed pork rinds

Directions:
1. Preheat oven to 360 °F.
2. Thoroughly blend zucchinis, capers, 1/2 of Parmesan cheese, garlic, cream cheese, bacon, and fontina cheese until finely united.
3. Shape the mixture into balls.
4. Store at a low temperature for three hrs.
5. Combine the remaining Parmesan cheese, pork rinds broken in a food processor, dill, black pepper, onion residue, poppy seeds, and salt in a container for mixing.
6. Coat the cheese ball in the Parmesan mixture by rolling it in it.
7. Bake for fifteen to twenty minutes, shaking the baking dish once, in a preheated oven at 350 degrees Fahrenheit.

Nutrition: *Calories: 227; Fat: 12.5g; Carbs:4.3 g; Fiber: 9.4g; Protein: 14.5g*

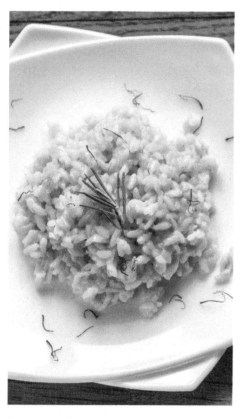

SWEET ORANGE AND LEMON BARLEY RISOTTO

Preparation Time: 5 minutes
Cooking time: 45 minutes
Servings: 4

Ingredients:

- 1 ½ cups barley pearls
- ¼ cup raisins
- 1 cup sweet orange, chopped, reserve juice
- 4 cups water
- 4 strips lemon peels
- ¼ cup white sugar, add more if needed

Directions:

1. Combine barley pearls, lemon peels, raisins, water, and white sugar into the Instant Pot Pressure Cooker.
2. Make sure the lid is securely fastened. Maintain the high pressure for the full ten minutes of cooking.
3. After hearing the buzzer, select the Quick Pressure Release option from the menu. This will result in a 7-minute depressurization. Take off the cover. Discard lemon peels.
4. Add in sweet orange and juices. Pour coconut cream. Allow residual heat cook the coconut cream. Adjust seasoning according to your preferred taste.
5. To serve, ladle equal amounts into dessert bowls. Cool slightly before serving.

Nutrition: *Calories: 124; Fat: 11g; Carbs: 3.9g; Fiber: 15g; Protein: 28g*

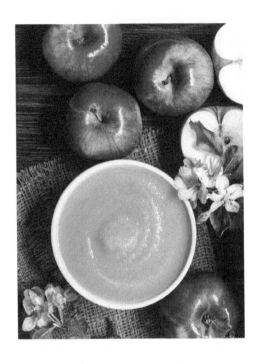

HOMEMADE APPLESAUCE

Preparation Time: 5 minutes
Cooking time: 45 minutes
Servings: 8

Ingredients:
- 10 soft-fleshed apples, quartered
- ¼ tsp. nutmeg powder
- 1 tsp. cinnamon powder
- ¼ cup sugar
- ¼ cup water

Directions:
1. Put the apples, nutmeg powder, cinnamon powder, sugar, and water into the pressure cooker that comes with the Instant Pot.
2. Make sure the lid is securely fastened. Cook for a total of 15 minutes at the highest possible pressure.
3. At the sound of the buzzer, select the option for the Quick Pressure Release. This will result in a 7-minute depressurization. Take off the cover.
4. Mash apples until the desired consistency is achieved. Adjust seasoning according to your preferred taste.
5. Spoon applesauce into bowls. Store leftovers in the fridge. This is best served cold.

Nutrition: *Calories: 345; Fat: 12g; Carbs: 3.4g; Fiber: 5g; Protein: 28g*

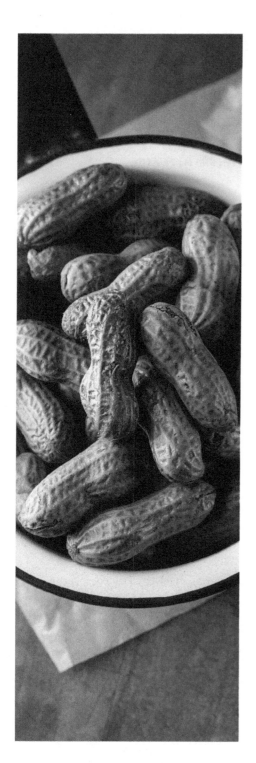

BOILED PEANUTS

Preparation Time: 5 minutes
Cooking time: 45 minutes
Servings: 4-6

Ingredients:
- 2 1/2 lbs. raw, unshelled peanuts
- 1 cup salt
- 4 cups water

Directions:
1. Place unshelled peanuts, salt, and water into the Instant Pot Pressure Cooker.
2. Lock the lid in place. Press the high pressure and cook for 10 minutes.
3. Once the beep sounds, Choose Natural Pressure Release. Depressurizing would take 20 minutes. Remove the lid.
4. Cool before pouring to a colander. Rinse well to remove most of the salt. Drain.
5. To serve, scoop just the right amount of peanuts into bowls. Shell peanuts as you eat.

Nutrition: *Calories: 132; Fat: 11g; Carbs: 1.4g; Fiber: 8g; Protein: 13g*

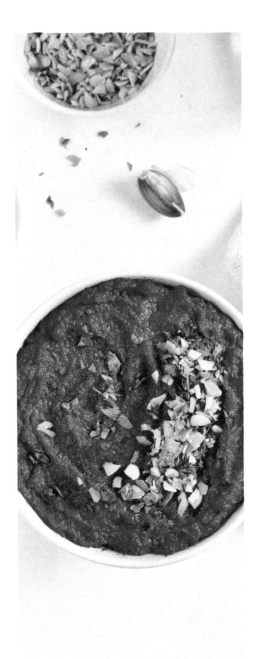

HOMEMADE BEET HUMMUS

Preparation Time: 5 minutes
Cooking time: 45 minutes
Servings: 8

Ingredients:

- 5 pieces cucumbers, thickly sliced
- 6 cups water
- 2 lbs. red beets, peeled
- 1 garlic clove, peeled
- 3 tbsp. tahini
- 3 tbsp. cumin powder
- 2 tbsp. Spanish paprika
- 3 Tbsp. lemon juice, freshly squeezed
- ¼ tsp. salt
- 1 tbsp. olive oil
- 1 tsp. white sesame seeds, toasted
- ¼ cup fresh cilantro, chopped

Directions:

1. Place water, red beets, and garlic clove into the Instant Pot Pressure Cooker.
2. Lock the lid in place. Press the high pressure and cook for 1 minute.
3. When the beep sounds, Choose the Quick Pressure Release. This will depressurize for 7 minutes. Remove the lid. Cool slightly before proceeding.
4. Discard solids but keep 1 cup of the cooking liquid.
5. Be sure to include the cooking liquid in the beets when you transfer them to an immersion blender. To season, add cumin powder, Spanish paprika, Spanish tahini, lemon juice, and salt to taste. To a smooth consistency, process. Make adjustments to the seasoning so that it meets your preferences.
6. Pour beet hummus into a bowl. Garnish with sesame seeds, cilantro, and olive oil. Serve with sliced cucumbers or crackers.
7. Store leftovers in the fridge. Use as needed.

Nutrition: *Calories: 154 ; Fat: 12g; Carbs: 1.9g; Fiber: 8g; Protein: 11g*

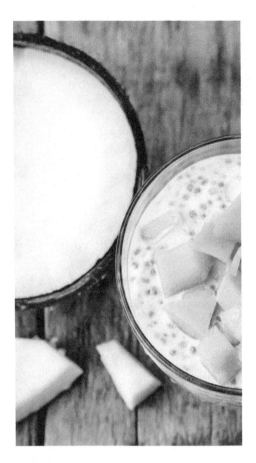

COCONUT PUDDING WITH TROPICAL FRUIT

Preparation Time: 15 minutes
Cooking time: 45 minutes
Servings: 4

Ingredients:

- ¼ lb. sticky rice balls
- 2 cups ripe plantains, sliced into thick disks
- 2 cans thick coconut cream, divided
- 1 cup taro, diced
- ½ cup tapioca pearls
- 1 cup sweet potato, diced
- 4 cups water
- 1 cup sugar
- Pinch of salt

Directions:

1. Combine sticky rice balls, taro, ripe plantains, tapioca pearls, water, white sugar, sweet potato, 1 can of coconut cream, and salt into the Instant Pot Pressure Cooker.
2. Make sure the lid is securely fastened. Maintain the high pressure for the full ten minutes of cooking.
3. At the sound of the buzzer, select the option for the Quick Pressure Release. This will result in a 7-minute depressurization. Take off the cover.
4. Tip in the remaining can of coconut cream. Allow residual heat to cook the coconut cream.
5. To serve, ladle equal amounts into dessert bowls.

Nutrition: *Calories: 213 ; Fat: 11g; Carbs: 2.7g; Fiber: 18gg; Protein: 21g*

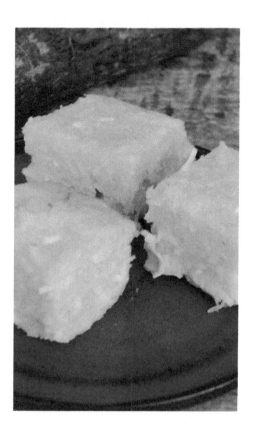

SWEET COCONUT CASSAVA

Preparation Time: 15 minutes
Cooking time: 1 minutes
Servings: 4

Ingredients:

- 2 lbs. yellow cassava, chopped into large chunks
- 1 cup white sugar
- 1 can thick coconut cream
- ¼ tsp. coconut oil
- 4 cups water
- 1/8 tsp. vanilla extract
- Pinch of salt

Directions:

1. Lightly grease the insides of the Instant Pot Pressure Cooker with coconut oil.
2. Pour water. Add in yellow cassava, sugar, and salt.
3. Lock the lid in place. Press the high pressure and cook for 7 minutes.
4. At the sound of the buzzer, select the option for the Quick Pressure Release. This will result in a 7-minute depressurization. Take off the cover.
5. Tip in coconut cream and vanilla extract. Allow residual heat to cook the last two ingredients. Adjust seasoning according to your preferred taste.
6. To serve, ladle equal amounts into dessert bowls.

Nutrition: *Calories: 345 ; Fat: 12g; Carbs: 2.9g; Fiber: 9gg; Protein: 29g*

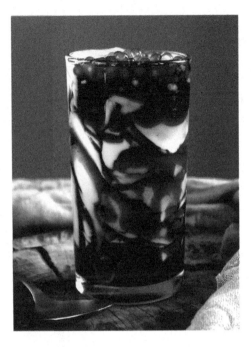

TOFU WITH SALTED CARAMEL PEARLS

Preparation Time: 5 minutes
Cooking time: 1 hour
Servings: 4

Ingredients:
- 1 cup tapioca pearls, no need to soak
- 2 packs 12 oz. soft silken tofu
- 5 cups water, divided
- 1 cup brown sugar
- 1/16 tsp. salt

Directions:
1. Pour tapioca pearls and water into the Instant Pot Pressure Cooker crockpot.
2. Lock the lid in place. Press the high pressure and cook for 10 minutes.
3. When the beep sounds, Choose Natural Pressure Release. Depressurizing would take 20 minutes. Remove the lid.
4. Reposition the lid and cook for another 5 minutes on high.
5. Once the beep sounds, Choose Natural Pressure Release. Depressurizing would take 20 minutes. Remove the lid. Pour out the contents of the pressure cooker over colander to drain.
6. Press the sauté button. Put back tapioca pearls to the crockpot. Add silken tofu, brown sugar, and salt.
7. Cook for 10 minutes or until the caramel thickens. Turn off the machine.
8. Meanwhile, scoop silken tofu into heat-resistant cups. Pour tapioca pearls and caramel on top. Serve.

Nutrition: *Calories: 125 ; Fat: 18g; Carbs: 1g; Fiber: 19g; Protein: 13g*

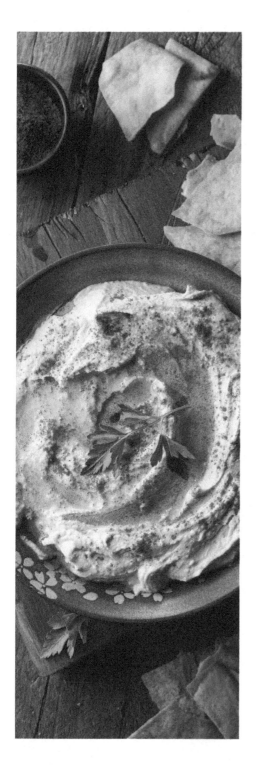

HOMEMADE HUMMUS

Preparation Time: 5 minutes
Cooking time: 1 hour
Servings: 4

Ingredients:

- 6 cups water
- 1 cup dry chickpeas
- 2 fresh bay leaves
- 4 garlic cloves, peeled
- 5 pieces crackers per person as base
- 3 tbsp. tahini
- 1/4tsp. cumin powder
- ½ cup lemon juice, freshly squeezed
- ¼ tsp. salt
- 1/16 tsp. toasted black sesame seeds
- 1/16 tsp. toasted white sesame seeds
- 1/16 tsp. red pepper flakes
- 2 tbsp. extra virgin olive oil
- 1 sprig of basil

Directions:

1. Place chickpeas, bay leaves, garlic cloves, and water into the Instant Pot Pressure Cooker.
2. Lock the lid in place. Press the high pressure and cook for 20 minutes.
3. Once the beep sounds, Choose Natural Pressure Release. Depressurizing would take 20 minutes. Remove the lid. Reserve 1 cup of cooking liquid. Discard the rest.
4. Transfer the cooked chickpeas and their cooking liquid to the container of an immersion blender. Add tahini, cumin powder, salt, and lemon juice to taste, then season with salt. To a smooth consistency, process. Make adjustments to the seasoning so that it meets your preferences.
5. Put the chickpeas in a bowl first. To finish, sprinkle the dish with toasted black and white sesame seeds, crushed red pepper, fresh basil, and olive oil. Accompany the dip with crackers.
6. Store leftovers in the fridge. Use as needed.

Nutrition: *Calories: 122 ; Fat: 11g; Carbs: 1.3g; Fiber: 21g; Protein: 13g*

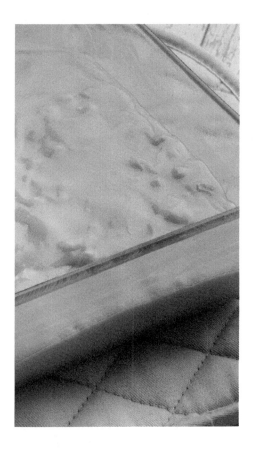

CORN COCONUT PUDDING

Preparation Time: 5minutes
Cooking time: 45 minutes
Servings: 3

Ingredients:
- 3 cups water
- 1 cup corn kernels
- ½ cup sticky rice
- ¼ cup ripe jackfruit, shredded
- ¼ tsp. vanilla extract
- ½ cup sugar
- 1/8 tsp. nutmeg powder
- 1/16 tsp. salt
- 2 cans thick coconut cream, divided

Directions:
1. Pour water, sticky rice, jackfruit, corn kernels, 1 can of coconut cream, nutmeg powder, vanilla extract, white sugar, and salt into the Instant Pot Pressure Cooker.
2. Make sure the lid is securely fastened. Cook for a total of seven minutes at a high pressure setting.
3. After hearing the buzzer, select the Quick Pressure Release option from the menu. This will result in a 7-minute depressurization. Take off the cover.
4. Tip in the remaining can of coconut cream. Allow residual heat cook the coconut cream. Adjust seasoning according to your preferred taste.
5. To serve, ladle equal amounts into dessert bowls.

Nutrition: *Calories: 213 ; Fat: 12g; Carbs: 2g; Fiber: 21g; Protein: 13g*

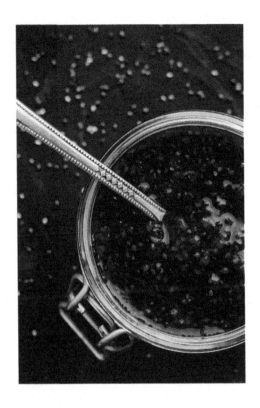

BERRY JAM WITH CHIA SEEDS

Preparation Time: 5 minutes
Cooking time: 45 minutes
Servings: 3

Ingredients:
- 2 cups fresh blueberries, stemmed
- 1 ½ cups water
- 1 cup fresh raspberries, stemmed
- 1 cup sugar
- 1/16 tsp. salt
- ½ cup chia seeds
- ¼ tbsp. lemon juice, freshly squeezed

Directions:
1. Place raspberries, blueberries, water, sugar, and salt into the Instant Pot Pressure Cooker. Stir.
2. Lock the lid in place. Press the high pressure and cook for 3 minutes.
3. Once the beep sounds, Choose the Quick Pressure Release. This will depressurize for 7 minutes. Remove the lid.
4. Add in chia seeds and lemon juice.
5. Using a potato masher, process the jam until it reaches the required consistency. You have the option of having your jam in either smooth or chunky form. After it has had time to cool, preserves should be stored in an airtight container. Use as needed.

Nutrition: *Calories: 128 ; Fat: 11g; Carbs: 4.8g; Fiber: 13g; Protein: 12g*

APPLE RISOTTO

Preparation Time: 5 minutes
Cooking time: 45 minutes
Servings: 3

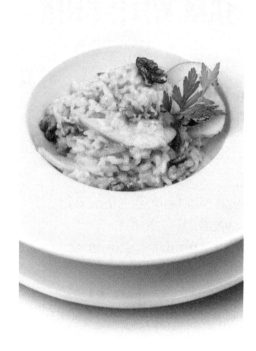

Ingredients:

- ½ cup apples, sliced into thick disks
- 1 ½ cups barley pearls
- ¼ tsp. cinnamon powder
- 2 cups water
- 1 cup apple juice
- 1 cup cashew milk
- ¼ cup cashew nuts, chopped
- 1/8 tsp. nutmeg powder
- ¼ cup sugar

Directions:

1. Place apples, apple juice, barley pearls, water, cinnamon powder, cashew nuts, cashew milk, nutmeg powder, and sugar inside the Instant Pot Pressure Cooker.
2. Make sure the lid is securely fastened. Cook for a total of seven minutes at a high pressure setting.
3. At the sound of the buzzer, select the option for the Quick Pressure Release. This will result in a 7-minute depressurization. Take off the cover. Make adjustments to the seasoning so that it meets your preferences.
4. To serve, ladle equal amounts into dessert bowls.

Nutrition: *Calories: 128 ; Fat: 11g; Carbs: 4.8g; Fiber: 13g; Protein: 12g*

CHAPTER THREE:

Breakfasts

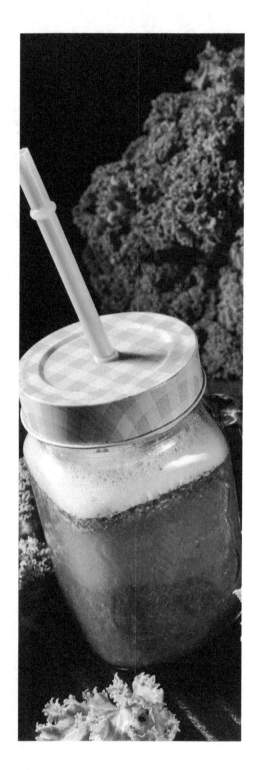

GUT-HEALING SMOOTHIE

Preparation Time: 5 minutes
Cooking time: 0 minutes
Servings: 4 smoothie glasses

Ingredients:

- 4 cups chopped organic kale
- 1 cup of organic mixed berries, frozen
- 1 teaspoon probiotic powder
- 2 teaspoons zinc carnosine
- 4 tablespoons grass-fed collagen protein powder
- 2 teaspoons deglycyrrhizinated licorice (DGL)
- 2 tablespoons coconut oil
- 2 tablespoons L-glutamine powder
- 2 cups almond milk, unsweetened

Directions:

1. Take a blender, add all the ingredients for smoothie in it, and pulse for 1 to 2 minutes until smooth.
2. Evenly divide the smoothie between four glasses and serve.

Nutrition: *Calories: 112.5 Cal; Fat: 8.4 g; Carbs: 4.8 g; Protein: 4.5 g; Fiber: 1.5 g*

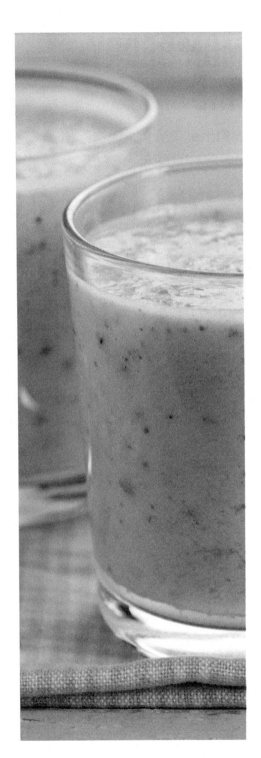

ALOE-MINT SMOOTHIE

Preparation Time: 5 minutes
Cooking time: 0 minutes
Servings: 4 smoothie glasses

Ingredients:
- 1 cup organic blueberries, frozen
- 2 tablespoons chia seeds
- 1/2 inch of organic ginger root
- 1 medium organic avocado, peeled, pitted, diced
- ¼ cup mint leaves
- 6 tablespoons collagen hydrolysate
- 4 tablespoons coconut oil
- 8 fluid ounces aloe vera juice
- 2 cups of coconut water

Directions:
1. Take a blender, add all the ingredients for smoothie in it, and pulse for 1 to 2 minutes until smooth.
2. Evenly divide the smoothie between four glasses and serve.

Nutrition: *Calories: 337 Cal; Fat: 20.6 g; Carbs: 17 g; Protein: 21.1 g; Fiber: 7.1 g*

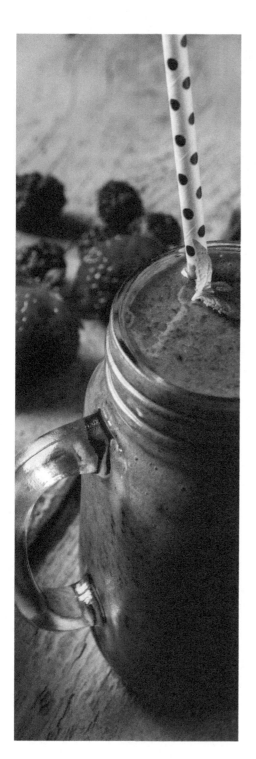

CINNAMON BERRY SMOOTHIE

Preparation Time: 5 minutes
Cooking time: 50 minutes
Servings: 4 smoothie glasses

Ingredients:

- 2 cups organic strawberries, frozen
- 2 cups organic kale
- ½ teaspoon cinnamon
- 1 medium organic avocado, pitted
- 10 drops vanilla extract, unsweetened
- 3 cups almond milk, unsweetened

Directions:

1. Take a blender, add all the ingredients for smoothie in it, and pulse for 1 to 2 minutes until smooth.
2. Evenly divide the smoothie between four glasses and serve.

Nutrition: *Calories: 113.5 Cal; Fat: 7.2 g; Carbs: 9.9 g; Protein: 2.3 g; Fiber: 4.3 g*

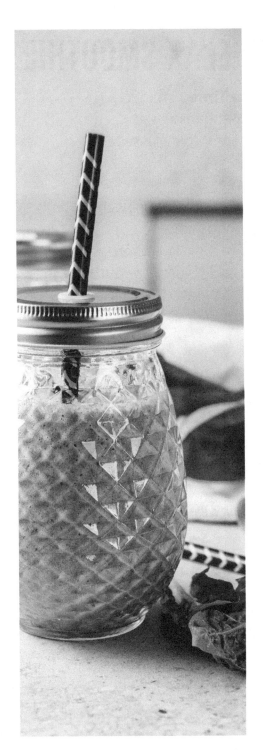

SPINACH AND ALOE SMOOTHIE

Preparation Time: 5 minutes
Cooking time: 0 minutes
Servings: 4 smoothie glasses

Ingredients:

- 4 cups fresh organic spinach
- 4 teaspoons vanilla extract, unsweetened
- 4 teaspoons cinnamon
- 2 cups Greek yogurt
- 4 fluid ounces aloe vera juice
- 2 cups almond milk, unsweetened

Directions:

1. Take a blender, add all the ingredients for smoothie in it, and pulse for 1 to 2 minutes until smooth.
2. Evenly divide the smoothie between four glasses and serve.

Nutrition: *Calories: 108 Cal; Fat: 2 g; Carbs: 8.6 g; Protein: 13.8 g; Fiber: 2.1 g*

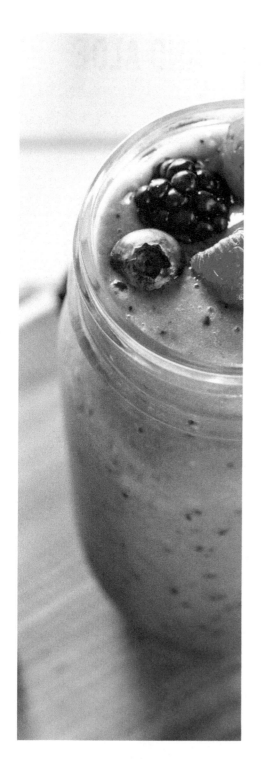

BERRY FLAX SMOOTHIE

Preparation Time: 5 minutes
Cooking time: 0 minutes
Servings: 4 smoothie glasses

Ingredients:

- 2 cups fresh organic spinach
- 2 tablespoons flax seeds, ground
- ½ cup of organic strawberries, frozen
- ½ cup organic blueberries, frozen
- 2 teaspoons grated organic ginger
- 4 cups almond milk, unsweetened

Directions:

1. Take a blender, add all the ingredients for smoothie in it, and pulse for 1 to 2 minutes until smooth.
2. Evenly divide the smoothie between four glasses and serve.

Nutrition: *Calories: 82 Cal; Fat: 4.4 g; Carbs: 8.2 g; Protein: 2.5 g; Fiber: 2.6 g*

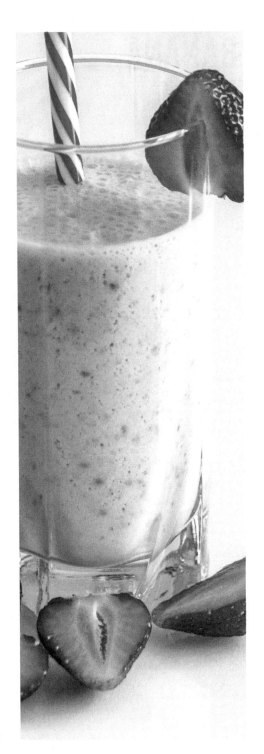

STRAWBERRY HEALTHY GUT SMOOTHIE

Preparation Time: 5 minutes
Cooking time: 0 minutes
Servings: 4 smoothie glasses

Ingredients:

- 2 cups organic romaine lettuce
- 1 cup organic strawberries, frozen
- 1 medium organic avocado, peeled, pitted, diced
- 2 cups organic kale
- 3 cups of coconut water

Directions:

1. Take a blender, add all the ingredients for smoothie in it, and pulse for 1 to 2 minutes until smooth.
2. Evenly divide the smoothie between four glasses and serve.

Nutrition: *Calories: 111.8 Cal; Fat: 5.5 g; Carbs: 13.4 g; Protein: 2.2 g; Fiber: 6 g*

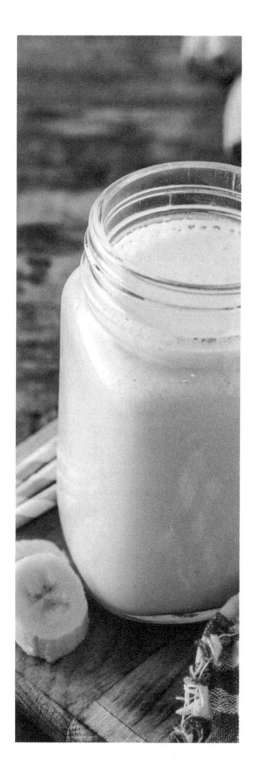

APPLE-BANANA SMOOTHIE

Preparation Time: 5 minutes
Cooking time: 0 minutes
Servings: 4 smoothie glasses

Ingredients:

- 20 walnuts
- 2 medium organic apple, cored, chopped
- 4 tablespoons chia seeds
- 2 medium organic banana, peeled, sliced
- 2 teaspoons cinnamon
- 3 cups Greek yogurt
- 2 cups of ice cubes
- 1 cup of water

Directions:

1. Take a blender, add all the ingredients for smoothie in it, and pulse for 1 to 2 minutes until smooth.
2. Evenly divide the smoothie between four glasses, sprinkle with additional cinnamon and serve.

Nutrition: *Calories: 389.3 Cal; Fat: 16.4 g; Carbs: 37 g; Protein: 23.4 g; Fiber: 8.5 g*

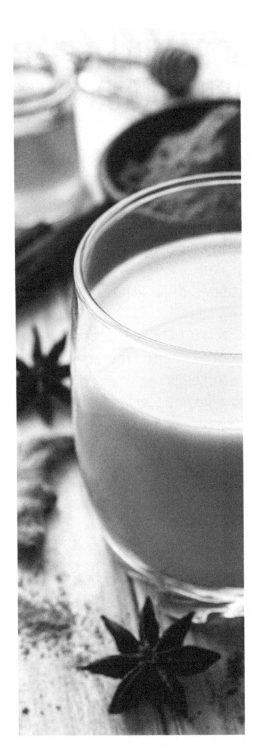

TURMERIC LATTE

Preparation Time: 5 minutes
Cooking time: 0 minutes
Servings: 4 glasses

Ingredients:

- 2-inch fresh organic ginger root, peeled, chopped
- 2 teaspoons ground turmeric
- 2 teaspoons ground cinnamon
- 2 teaspoons raw honey
- 4 cups coconut milk, unsweetened

Directions:

1. Take a blender, add all the ingredients for smoothie in it, and pulse for 1 to 2 minutes until smooth.
2. Evenly divide the smoothie between four glasses and serve.

Nutrition: *Calories: 62.8 Cal; Fat: 4.3 g; Carbs: 5.5 g; Protein: 0.6 g; Fiber: 1.4 g*

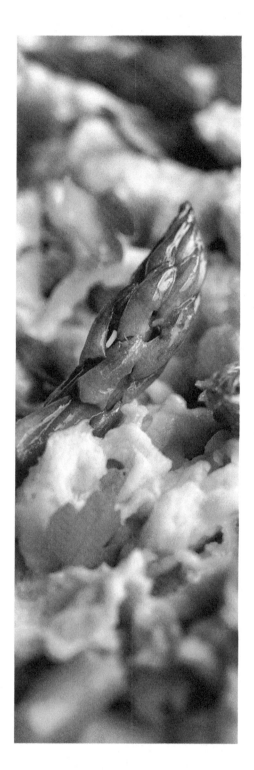

HERB SCRAMBLED EGG WITH ASPARAGUS

Preparation Time: 5 minutes
Cooking time: 10 minutes
Servings: 4 plates

Ingredients:

- 7 ounces organic asparagus spears, peeled, scaled
- ½ cup chopped organic tarragon
- ½ teaspoon salt
- ½ teaspoon ground black pepper
- 4 tablespoons unsalted butter
- 8 pasteurized eggs
- Grated cottage cheese, for topping
- Slices of sourdough bread, toasted
- ½ cup of water

Directions:

1. Rinse the asparagus thoroughly, then peel and scale them and cut into bite-size pieces.
2. Take an ovenproof casserole dish, pour in water, add asparagus in layers, and cover the top with a plastic wrap.
3. Make holes in the plastic wrap by poking fork in it and then microwave asparagus for 4 to 5 minutes until done, checking asparagus every 2 minutes.
4. When done, remove the casserole dish from the oven, remove the plastic wrap, transfer asparagus to a plate, and set aside until required.
5. Prepare the scrambled eggs and for this, take a large skillet pan, add butter and let it melt until it starts to melts.
6. Crack the eggs in a bowl, whisk until blended, then pour the eggs into the pan and cook the eggs until scrambled to desire level.
7. Season eggs with salt and black pepper, add tarragon, stir well and remove the pan from heat.
8. Evenly divide asparagus between four plates, top them evenly with scrambled eggs, sprinkle with cheese, and serve with a toast of sourdough bread.

Nutrition: *Calories: 210 Cal; Fat: 14 g; Carbs: 1 g; Protein: 21 g; Fiber: 0 g*

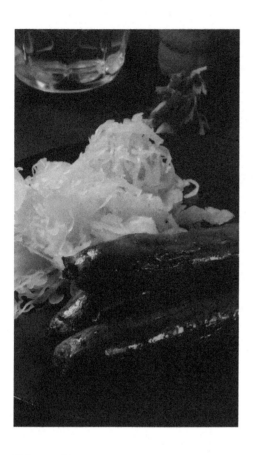

SAUSAGE AND SAUERKRAUT

Preparation Time: 5 minutes
Cooking time: 20 minutes
Servings: 4 plates

Ingredients:

- 8 grass-fed beef sausages, uncured
- 2 medium organic white onion, peeled, sliced
- 2 medium organic apples, cored, sliced
- 4 cups organic sauerkraut
- 1 teaspoon ground black pepper
- ½ teaspoon caraway seeds
- 4 tablespoons unsalted butter
- 1 cup sauerkraut liquid

Directions:

1. Take a large skillet pan, place it over medium-low heat, add butter and when it melts, add onions and cook for 5 minutes until softened.
2. Switch heat to the low level, sprinkle black pepper and caraway seeds over onions, add sauerkraut, pour in sauerkraut liquid, stir until mixed and simmer for 20 minutes, covering the pan.
3. Meanwhile, take a grilling pan, place it over medium heat, grease it with coconut oil and when hot, add sausages and cook for 15 to 20 minutes until thoroughly cooked, turning every 5 minutes.
4. When sausages have cooked, let them rest for 5 minutes and then divide them into four plates, two sausages per plate.
5. Add sauerkraut mixture, then add some apple slices and serve.

Nutrition: *Calories: 351.5 Cal; Fat: 23 g; Carbs: 26.4 g; Protein: 9.7 g; Fiber: 9.8 g*

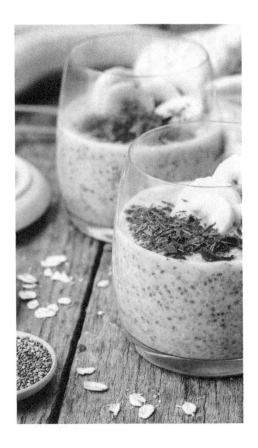

BANANA, FLAX AND TURMERIC OATS

Preparation Time: 4 hours and 5 minutes
Cooking time: 0 minutes
Servings: 4 bowls

Ingredients:

- ½ cup ground flaxseed
- 4 small organic bananas, peeled
- 2 cups rolled oats
- 4 teaspoons ground turmeric
- 2 teaspoons ground cinnamon
- 2 cups almond milk, unsweetened
- ½ cup Greek yogurt
- 2 cups of water
- Raspberries for serving

Directions:

1. Take a jar or container, add flaxseeds, oats, turmeric, and cinnamon and stir until mixed.
2. Place bananas in a shallow dish, mash well with a fork and then add to the oats mixture.
3. Add yogurt, pour in water and milk, stir until well combined, pour the mixture over fruits and oats and refrigerate for a minimum of 4 hours or overnight.
4. When ready to eat, evenly divide them between four bowls, top with berries or any other favorite toppings and serve.

Nutrition: *Calories: 419.3 Cal; Fat: 16.3 g; Carbs: 58.7 g; Protein: 9.4 g; Fiber: 12.3 g*

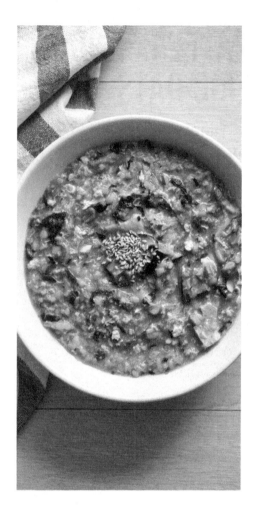

SWEET MISO PORRIDGE

Preparation Time: 10 minutes
Cooking time: 10 minutes
Servings: 4 bowls

Ingredients:

For Porridge:
- 4 cups rolled porridge oats
- 1/2 teaspoons ground ginger
- 1 tablespoon chia seeds
- 1 tablespoon white sweet miso
- 1/2 teaspoon vanilla powder
- 2 cardamom pods
- 8 cups almond milk

For Topping:
- 4 medium organic banana, peeled, sliced
- 4 medium organic pears, diced
- ½ cup pecan nuts
- 4 tablespoons raw honey

Directions:
1. Prepare the porridge and for this, take a medium saucepan, place it over medium-high heat, add chia seeds, oats, and ginger and pour in the milk.
2. Crush the seeds of cardamom, add to the porridge, stir well and cook for 8 to 10 minutes until oats have cooked, and most of the liquid is absorbed.
3. Remove pan from heat, add vanilla powder and miso paste, stir well and then evenly divide porridge between four bowls.
4. Top evenly with banana, pear, nuts, and honey and serve straight away.

Nutrition: *Calories: 1285 Cal; Fat: 31.4 g; Carbs: 221.7 g; Protein: 29 g; Fiber: 30 g*

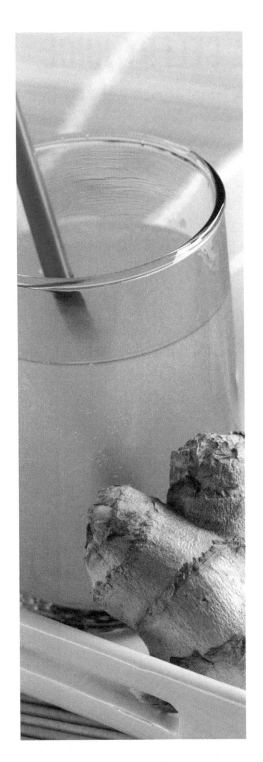

FRUITY GINGER JUICE

Preparation Time: 10 minutes
Cooking time: 0 minutes
Servings: 2

Ingredients:
- 2 apples, cored and unevenly sliced
- 2 pears, cored and unevenly sliced
- 2 kiwi fruits, halved
- 1 (¾-inch) portion fresh ginger, skinned and chopped
- ½-¾ C. clean water

Directions:
1. Put all of the ingredients together into a powerful blender, and whir them around until they are thoroughly mixed.
2. Through a cheesecloth-lined sieve, strain the juice and pour it into two glasses.
3. Immediately serve after preparing the drinks.

Nutrition: *Calories: 293; Fat: 1.3g; Carbs: 75.7g; Fiber: 14.5g; Protein: 2.5g*

PEAR & CELERY JUICE

Preparation Time: 10 minutes
Cooking time: 0 minutes
Servings: 2

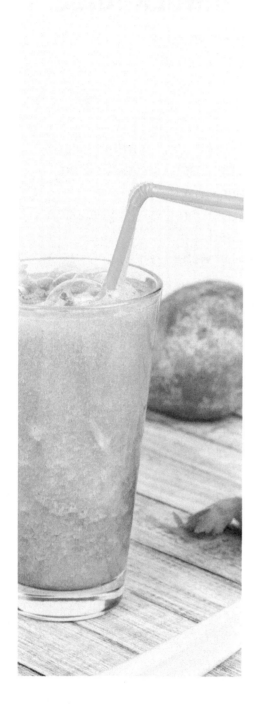

Ingredients:

- 4 large pears
- 4 celery stalks
- 1 teaspoon honey
- half C. clean water

Directions:

1. Put all of the ingredients into the bread maker in the direction that is suggested by the creator of the bread machine.
2. Run the dough through the cycle for sweet bread or whole-wheat flour. Put all of the ingredients together into a powerful blender, and whir them around until they are thoroughly mixed.
3. Use a cheesecloth-lined sieve to strain the juice and pour in two glasses.
4. Immediately serve after preparing the drinks.

Nutrition: *Calories: 258; Fat: 0.7g; Carbs: 67.6g; Fiber: 13.5g; Protein: 1.8g*

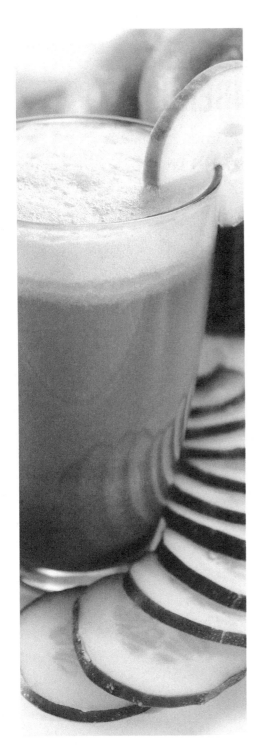

APPLE & CUCUMBER JUICE

Preparation Time: 10 minutes
Cooking time: 0 minutes
Servings: 2

Ingredients:

- 2 cucumbers unevenly cut and split
- 4 green apples, cored and sectioned
- 1 lemon, halved
- 1 C. clean water

Directions:

1. Put all of the ingredients together into a powerful blender, and whir them around until they are thoroughly mixed.
2. Through a cheesecloth-lined sieve, strain the juice and pour into two glasses.
3. Immediately serve after preparing the drinks.

Nutrition: *Calories: 279; Fat: 0.4g; Carbs: 73.2g; Fiber: 12.5g; Protein: 3.2g*

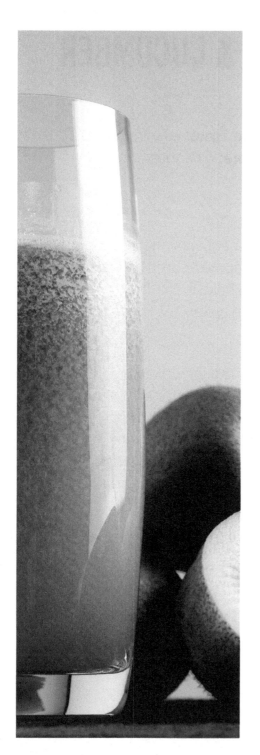

KIWI, APPLE & CUCUMBER JUICE

Preparation Time: 10 minutes
Cooking time: 0 minutes
Servings: 2

Ingredients:
- 4 kiwi fruit, skinned
- 3 Granny Smith apples, cored and divided
- 1 large cucumber, unevenly cut

Directions:
1. Put all of the components into the juicer, and then extract the juice using the procedure recommended by the manufacturer.
2. After straining it through a strainer lined with cheesecloth, divide the juice evenly between two glasses.
3. Immediately serve after preparing the drinks.

Nutrition: *Calories: 289; Fat: 1.6g; Carbs: 73.9g; Fiber: 13.4g; Protein: 3.6g*

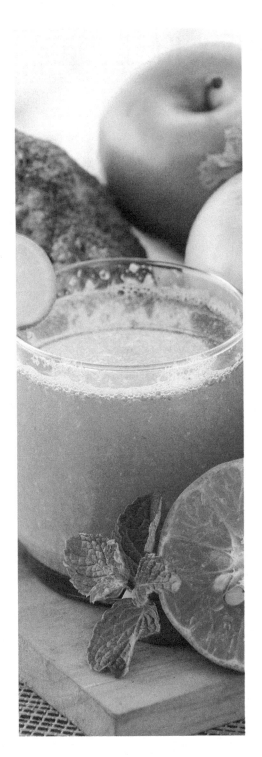

BROCCOLI, APPLE & ORANGE JUICE

Preparation Time: 10 minutes
Cooking time: 0 minutes
Servings: 2

Ingredients:
- 2 broccoli stalks, sliced
- 2 large green apples, cored and divided
- 3 large oranges, peeled and sectioned
- 4 tbsp. fresh parsley

Directions:
1. Put all of the components into the juicer, and then extract the juice using the procedure recommended by the manufacturer.
2. Through a cheesecloth-lined strainer, strain the juice and transfer into 2 glasses.
3. Immediately Serve after preparing the drinks.

Nutrition: *Calories: 254; Fat: 0.8g; Carbs: 64.7g; Fiber: 12.7g; Protein: 3.8g*

ORANGE & KALE JUICE

Preparation Time: 10 minutes
Cooking time: 0 minutes
Servings: 2

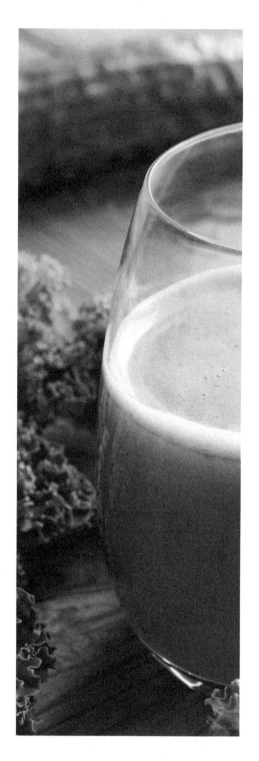

Ingredients:
- 5 large oranges, skinned, and sectioned
- 2 bunches fresh kale

Directions:
1. Put all of the components into the juicer, and then extract the juice using the procedure recommended by the manufacturer.
2. Through a cheesecloth-lined strainer, strain the juice and transfer into 2 glasses.
3. Immediately serve after preparing the drinks.

Nutrition: *Calories: 315; Fat: 0.6g; Carbs: 75.1g; Fiber: 14g; Protein: 10.3g*

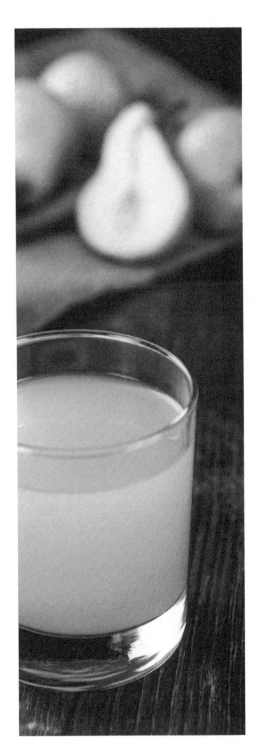

PEAR & FENNEL JUICE

Preparation Time: 10 minutes
Cooking time: 0 minutes
Servings: 2

Ingredients:
- 3 pears, cored, and quartered
- 3 C. raw kale
- 1 fennel bulb
- 1 (½-inch) quantity of fresh ginger, skinned

Directions:
1. Put all of the components into the juicer, and then extract the juice using the procedure recommended by the manufacturer.
2. Through a cheesecloth-lined strainer, strain the juice and transfer into 2 glasses.
3. Serve immediately.

Nutrition: *Calories: 270; Fat: 0.7g; Carbs: 67.4g; Fiber: 15g; Protein: 5.7g*

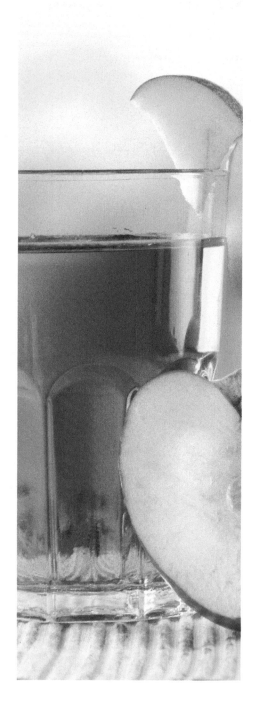

APPLE, ORANGE & SWISS CHARD JUICE

Preparation Time: 10 minutes
Cooking time: 0 minutes
Servings: 2

Ingredients:
- 3 C. Swiss chard
- 3 apples, cored and quartered
- 2 oranges, peeled and sectioned

Directions:
1. Put all of the ingredients together into the juicer, and then extract the juice using the procedure recommended by the manufacturer.
2. Through a cheesecloth-lined strainer, strain the juice and transfer into 2 glasses.
3. Immediately serve after preparing the drinks.

Nutrition: *Calories: 271; Fat: 1g; Carbs: 69.8g; Fiber: 13.4g; Protein: 3.6g*

CARROT, BEET & APPLE JUICE

Preparation Time: 10 minutes
Cooking time: 0 minutes
Servings: 2

Ingredients:
- 3 large carrots, skinned, and sliced
- 3 medium red beetroots, clipped, skinned, and sliced
- 1 large red apple, cored, and divided
- 1 large green apple, cored, and divided

Directions:
1. Put all of the ingredients together into the juicer, and then extract the juice using the procedure recommended by the manufacturer.
2. Through a cheesecloth-lined strainer, strain the juice and transfer into 2 glasses.
3. Immediately serve after preparing the drinks.

Nutrition: *Calories: 284; Fat: 0.9g; Carbs: 71.8g; Fiber: 13.8g; Protein: 4.3g*

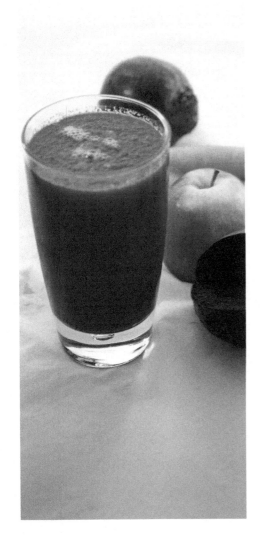

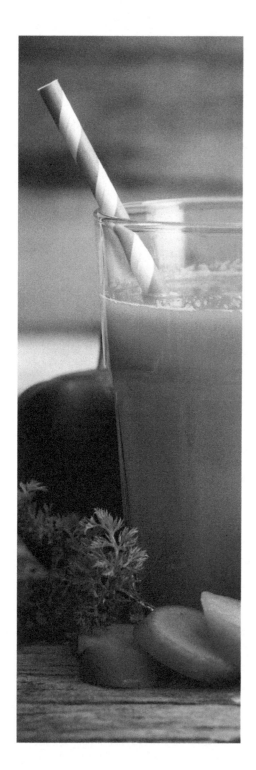

APPLE, PEAR & CARROT JUICE

Preparation Time: 10 minutes
Cooking time: 0 minutes
Servings: 2

Ingredients:

- 2 medium sized apples, cored and divided
- 2 medium sized pears, cored and divided
- 4 large carrots, peeled and roughly chopped
- 4 celery stalks

Directions:

1. Put all of the ingredients together into the juicer, and then extract the juice using the procedure recommended by the manufacturer.
2. Through a cheesecloth-lined strainer, strain the juice and transfer into 2 glasses.
3. Immediately serve after preparing the drinks.

Nutrition: *Calories: 292; Fat: 0.8g; Carbs: 75.6g; Fiber: 15.4g; Protein: 2.6g*

APPLE, PEAR & ORANGE JUICE

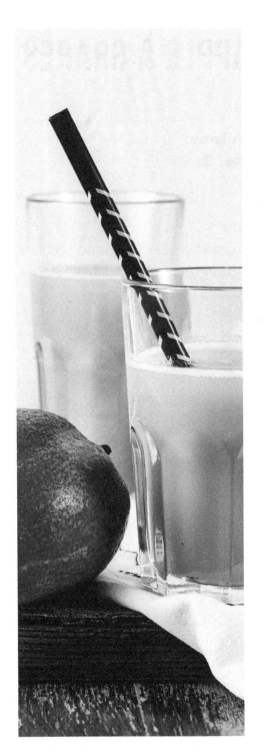

Preparation Time: 10 minutes
Cooking time: 0 minutes
Servings: 2

Ingredients:

- 4 apples, cored, and divided
- 4 pears, cored, and quartered
- 2 oranges, peeled, seeded, and sectioned
- 6 celery stalks

Directions:

1. Put all of the ingredients together into the juicer, and then extract the juice using the procedure recommended by the manufacturer.
2. After straining it through a strainer lined with cheesecloth, divide the juice evenly between two glasses.
3. Immediately serve after preparing the drinks.

Nutrition: *Calories: 568; Fat: 1.7g; Carbs: 128.7g; Fiber: 29g; Protein: 4.8g*

KIWI, APPLE & GRAPES JUICE

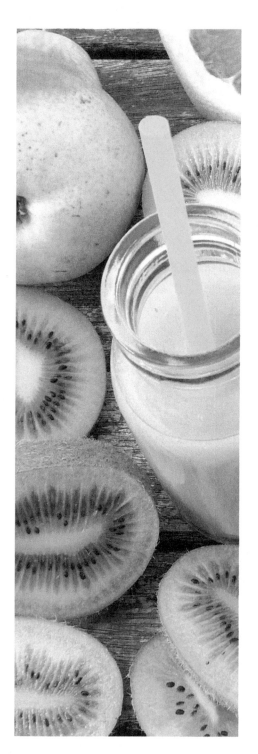

Preparation Time: 10 minutes
Cooking time: 0 minutes
Servings: 2

Ingredients:
- 3 large sized kiwis, skinned, and sliced
- 3 large sized green apples, cored, and sectioned
- 2 C. seedless green grapes
- 2 teaspoon raw lime juice

Directions:
1. Put all of the ingredients together into the juicer, and then extract the juice using the procedure recommended by the manufacturer.
2. After straining it through a strainer lined with cheesecloth, divide the juice evenly between two glasses.
3. Immediately serve after preparing the drinks.

Nutrition: *Calories: 304; Fat: 2.2g; Carbs: 79g; Fiber: 12.5g; Protein: 6.2g*

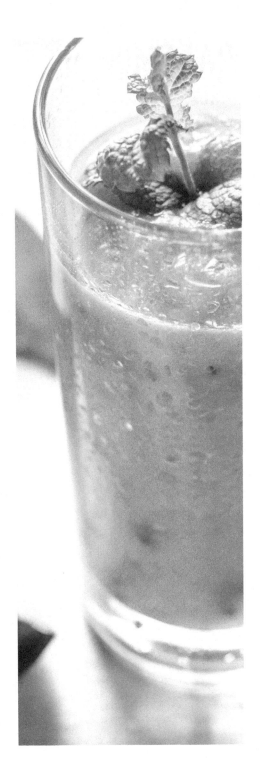

PEACH & OAT SMOOTHIE

Preparation Time: 10 minutes
Cooking time: 0 minutes
Servings: 2

Ingredients:
- 2 cups of frozen peaches, pitted
- ½ of rolled oats
- ¼ teaspoon of ground cinnamon
- 1 and ½ of plain yogurt
- ½ of fresh orange Juice

Directions:
1. Put all of the ingredients together into a powerful blender, and whir them around until they become creamy.
2. The smoothie should be served immediately in two glasses, and you should pour it in.

Nutrition: *Calories: 328; Fat: 4.1g; Carbs: 56g; Fiber: 5g; Protein: 15g*

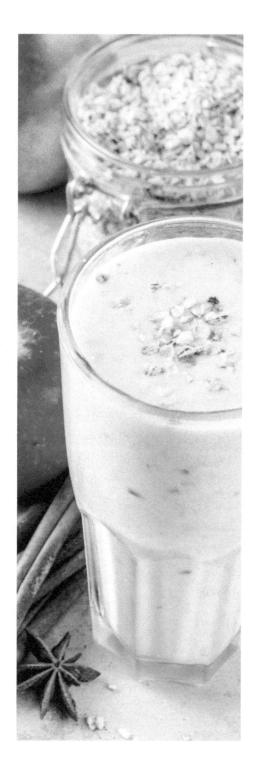

APPLE OAT SMOOTHIE

Preparation Time: 10 minutes
Cooking time: 0 minutes
Servings: 4

Ingredients:

- 2 ounces of rolled oats
- 4 apples, skinned, cored, and sliced unevenly
- 4 scoops unsweetened protein powder
- 1 teaspoon stevia powder
- 1 teaspoon ground cinnamon
- 1 teaspoon ground nutmeg
- 17 ounces plain yogurt
- 2 cups of milk

Directions:

1. Put all of the ingredients together into a powerful blender, and whir them around until they become creamy.
2. After pouring the smoothie into the glasses, it should be served right away.

Nutrition: *Calories: 437; Fat: 6.6g; Carbs: 55.6g; Fiber: 7.3g; Protein: 38.7g*

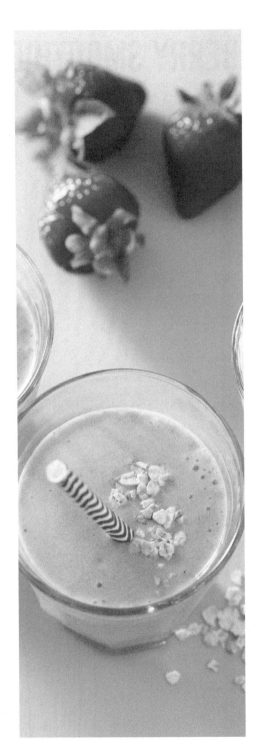

STRAWBERRY OAT SMOOTHIE

Preparation Time: 10 minutes
Cooking time: 0 minutes
Servings: 2

Ingredients:

- 1½ cup frozen strawberries
- 1 medium banana, skinned and cut
- ¼ C. old-fashioned oats
- 1 C. fat-free plain yogurt
- ¾ C. unsweetened almond milk

Directions:

1. Put all of the ingredients together into a powerful blender, and whir them around until they become creamy.
2. The smoothie should be served immediately in two glasses, and you should pour it in.

Nutrition: *Calories: 227; Fat: 4g; Carbs: 37.9g; Fiber: 6.1g; Protein: 10g*

BLACKBERRY SMOOTHIE

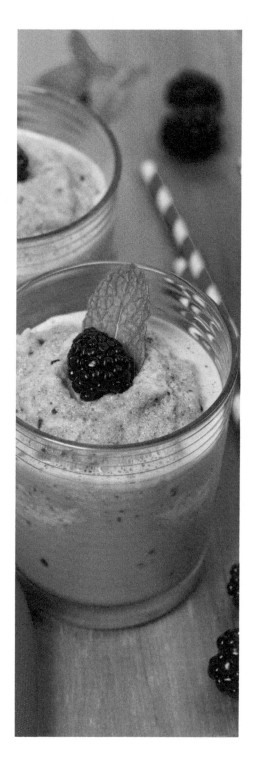

Preparation Time: 10 minutes
Cooking time: 0 minutes
Servings: 2

Ingredients:

- 2 cups frozen blackberries
- 1 small banana, skinned and cut
- 2 tablespoons raw lime juice
- 1 tablespoon honey
- 1 teaspoon lime zest, peeved
- ½ cup fat-free simple yogurt
- 1 cup light coconut milk

Directions:

1. Put all of the ingredients together into a powerful blender, and whir them around until they become creamy.
2. The smoothie should be served immediately in two glasses, and you should pour it in.

Nutrition: *Calories: 259; Fat: 7.6g; Carbs: 44.6g; Fiber: 10.1g; Protein: 6.1g*

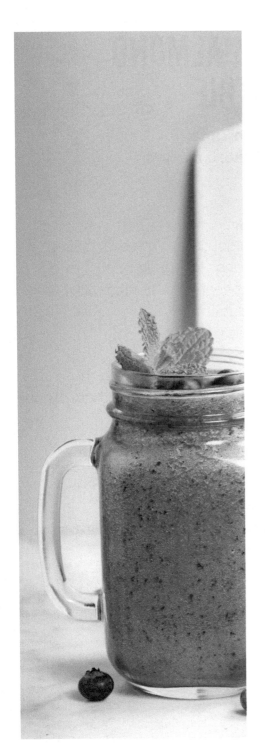

BLUEBERRY & AVOCADO SMOOTHIE

Preparation Time: 10 minutes
Cooking time: 0 minutes
Servings: 2

Ingredients:
- 2 cups raw blueberries
- 1 large banana, skinned and cut
- 1 small avocado, skinned, eroded and sliced
- 1 C. fresh cranberry juice
- ¼ C. ice cubes

Directions:
1. Put all of the ingredients together into a powerful blender, and whir them around until they become creamy.
2. The smoothie should be served immediately in two glasses, and you should pour it in.

Nutrition: *Calories: 304; Fat: 12g; Carbs: 47.9g; Fiber: 12.3g; Protein: 3.7g*

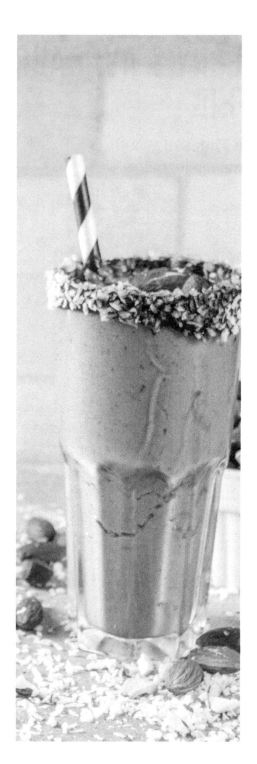

DATE & ALMOND SMOOTHIE

Preparation Time: 10 minutes
Cooking time: 0 minutes
Servings: 2

Ingredients:

- 1 C. Medjool dates, rutted, and sliced
- ½ C. almonds, chopped
- 1½ C. unsweetened almond milk
- ¼ C. ice cubes

Directions:

1. Put all of the ingredients together into a powerful blender, and whir them around until they become creamy.
2. The smoothie should be served immediately in two glasses, and you should pour it in.

Nutrition: *Calories: 418; Fat: 14.9g; Carbs: 73.4g; Fiber: 10.8g; Protein: 8g*

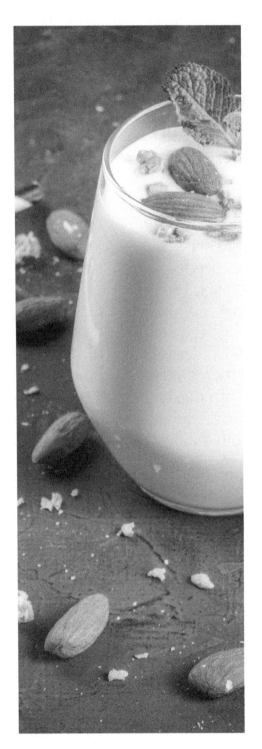

PEAR & ALMOND SMOOTHIE

Preparation Time: 10 minutes
Cooking time: 0 minutes
Servings: 2

Ingredients:

- 3 large pears, skinned, cored, and cut
- 2 tbsp. almonds, chopped
- ¼ teaspoon vanilla extract
- 1½ cup unsweetened almond milk
- ¼ cup ice cubes

Directions:

1. Put all of the ingredients together into a powerful blender, and whir them around until they become creamy.
2. The smoothie should be served immediately in two glasses, and you should pour it in.

Nutrition: *Calories: 247; Fat: 6g; Carbs: 50.6g; Fiber: 11.2g; Protein: 3.1g*

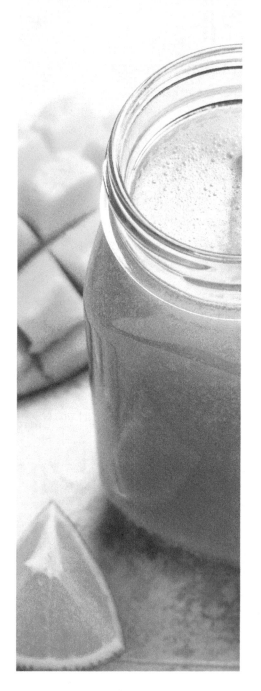

MANGO, ORANGE & CUCUMBER SMOOTHIE

Preparation Time: 10 minutes
Cooking time: 0 minutes
Servings: 2

Ingredients:
- ½ C. mango masses
- 2 oranges, skinned
- 2 C. cucumber, sliced
- 2 C. spinach

Directions:
1. Put all of the ingredients together into a powerful blender, and whir them around until they become creamy.
2. The smoothie should be served immediately in two glasses, and you should pour it in.

Nutrition: *Calories: 369; Fat: 5.9g; Carbs: 72.3g; Fiber: 14.7g; Protein: 11.9g*

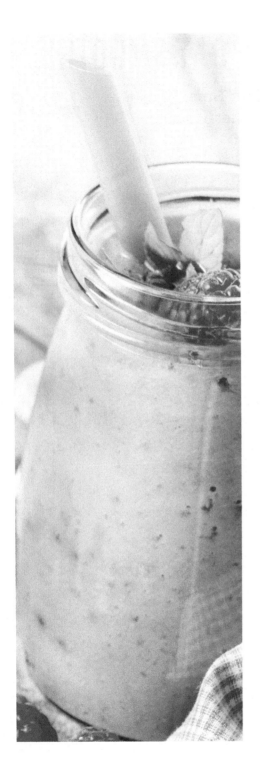

RASPBERRY OAT SMOOTHIE

Preparation Time: 10 minutes
Cooking time: 0 minutes
Servings: 2

Ingredients:

- 1¼ C. raw raspberries
- 2 bananas, skinned and cut
- ½ C. oats
- 1 scoop unsweetened protein powder
- 1 tablespoon maple syrup
- 1½ C. unsweetened almond milk
- ¼ C. ice cubes

Directions:

1. Put all of the ingredients together into a powerful blender, and whir them around until they become creamy.
2. The smoothie should be served immediately in two glasses, and you should pour it in.

Nutrition: *Calories: 337; Fat: 5.4g; Carbs: 58.2g; Fiber: 10.9g; Protein: 18.3g*

KIWI & OAT SMOOTHIE

Preparation Time: 10 minutes
Cooking time: 0 minutes
Servings: 2

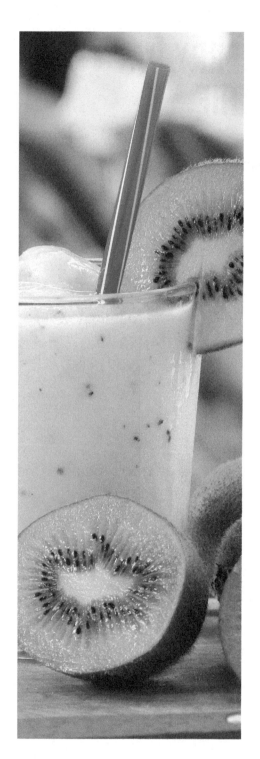

Ingredients:

- 4 kiwi fruits, skinned
- 2 bananas, skinned, and cut
- 6 tablespoons oats
- ½ teaspoon. fresh ginger, skinned, and cut
- 1 teaspoon maple syrup
- ¾ cup yogurt
- 1¼ cup unsweetened almond milk

Directions:

1. Put all of the ingredients together into a powerful blender, and whir them around until they become creamy.
2. The smoothie should be served immediately in two glasses, and you should pour it in.

Nutrition: *Calories: 357; Fat: 5.5g; Carbs: 69g; Fiber: 10g; Protein: 10.9g*

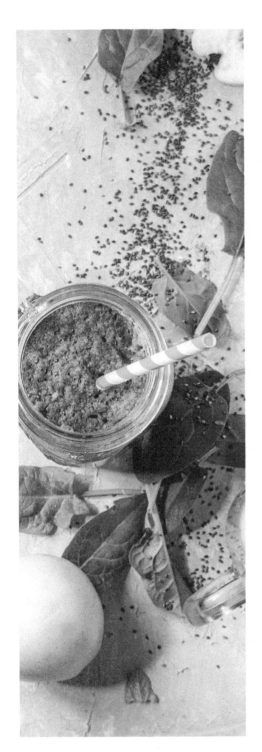

APPLE & SPINACH SMOOTHIE

Preparation Time: 10 minutes
Cooking time: 0 minutes
Servings: 2

Ingredients:

- 2 medium apples, skinned, cored, and cut
- 1 banana, skinned, and cut
- 3 cups raw spinach
- 1 scoop unsweetened protein powder
- 1 cup coconut water
- ¾ cup ice

Directions:

1. Put all of the ingredients together into a powerful blender, and whir them around until they become creamy.
2. The smoothie should be served immediately in two glasses, and you should pour it in.

Nutrition: *Calories: 279; Fat: 4.5g; Carbs: 50.5g; Fiber: 9.6g; Protein: 14.9g*

CUCUMBER & CELERY SMOOTHIE

Preparation Time: 10 minutes
Cooking time: 0 minutes
Servings: 2

Ingredients:
- 1 cucumber around 4 inches
- 1 celery trunk
- 1 romaine lettuce leaf
- 1 full lime, skinned
- 1 teaspoon ginger powder
- Tweak of ground turmeric
- 1 cup of water
- 1 cup of ice

Directions:
1. Put all of the ingredients together into a powerful blender, and whir them around until they become creamy.
2. The smoothie should be served immediately in two glasses, and you should pour it in.

Nutrition: *Calories: 138; Fat: 0.3g; Carbs: 29.8g; Fiber: 12.1g; Protein: 5.7g*

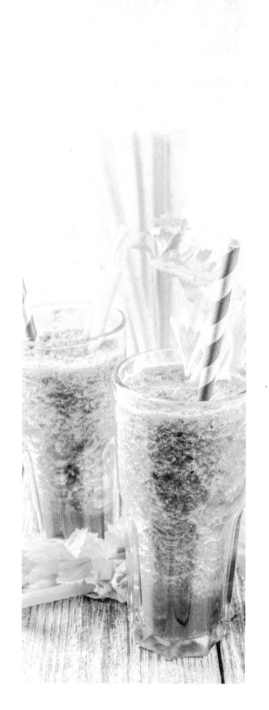

CHAPTER FOUR:
Lunches

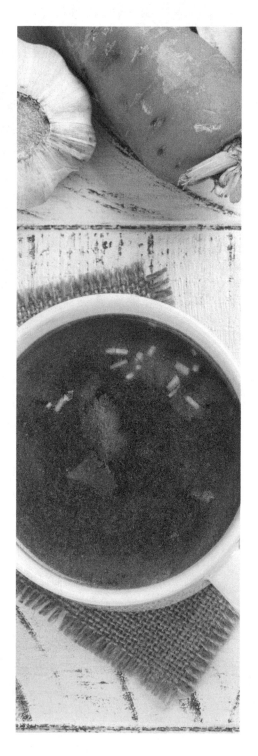

MUSHROOM & BEEF BONE BROTH

Preparation Time: 45 minutes
Cooking time: 37 hours
Servings: 2 to 3 quarts

Ingredients:

- 3 pounds mixed beef bones, ideally including marrow bones
- ½ cup dried porcini mushrooms
- 2 large carrots
- 1 large onion
- 2 celery stalks
- 1 dried bay leaf
- 2 tbsp apple cider vinegar (I use Bragg's)
- 4 quarts water, plus more if needed

Directions:

1. This is easiest to make in a large slow cooker (about 6 quarts). However, a large stock pot will do just fine—you will just have to keep an eye on it.
2. Preheat the oven to 400°F.
3. Place the bones on a baking sheet and roast for 30 minutes, until browned.
4. Roughly chop your mushrooms, carrots, onion, and celery.
5. Put the browned bones in the slow cooker or pot with the chopped veggies and the bay leaf and vinegar, and cover with the water.
6. Set your slow cooker on Low and cook for 36 hours. If using a pot, keep the heat very low and cover with a lid. Check the liquid level periodically, and add more water if too much is evaporating.
7. After 36 hours of simmering, remove the bones and place in a colander over a large bowl to catch the juices.
8. Pour the broth through a strainer into a large bowl. You will need to do this in batches, as the strainer fills up and needs to be emptied.
9. Discard the bones and vegetables. They are no longer nutritious—all the nutrients are in the broth.
10. Transfer the broth into mason jars for storage in the fridge or measure into freezer-safe containers or zip-top bags to store in the freezer.

Nutrition: *Calories: 20; Total fat: 0g; Saturated fat: 0g; Sodium: 0mg; Carbohydrates: 1g; Fiber: 0g; Protein: 5g*

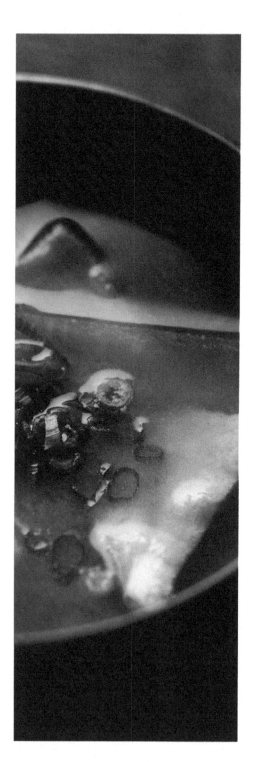

SHIITAKE-MISO COD SOUP

Preparation Time: 10 minutes
Cooking time: 25 minutes
Servings: 2

Ingredients:

- 2 pieces fresh cod, about ½ pound total
- 1 tablespoon coconut oil
- 1 onion, sliced thinly
- 1 garlic clove, minced
- 1 inch fresh ginger root, peeled
- 4 or 5 fresh shiitake mushrooms, sliced thinly
- 16 ounces bone broth bone broth (homemade, , or store-bought organic)
- 2 tablespoons gluten-free miso paste (I like Miso Master gluten-free brown rice)

Directions:

1. Cut the cod into bite-size pieces.
2. In a big saucepan over medium heat, heat the coconut oil. Add the onion, garlic, and ginger, and sauté until the onion is translucent, 3 to 4 minutes.
3. Add the mushrooms, and sauté for 10 minutes, or until the mushrooms are tender.
4. Add the bone broth, and bring to a boil.
5. Add the miso paste, and stir until it has melted and fully incorporated into the soup.
6. Bring to a boil. Add the fish, and cook for 5 minutes, then turn off the heat and let poach for another 1 to 2 minutes.

Nutrition: *Calories: 259; Total fat: 9g; Saturated fat: 6g; Sodium: 1,056mg; Carbohydrates: 17g; Fiber: 4g; Protein: 29g*

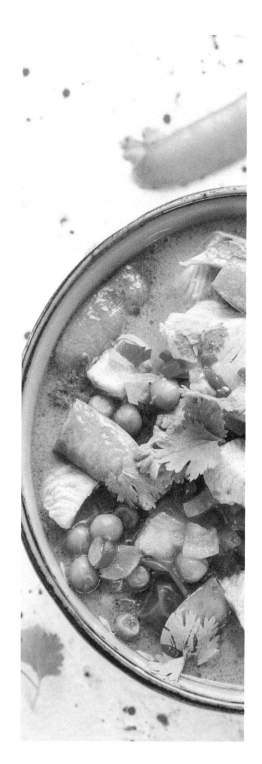

VEGETABLE-COCONUT CURRY SOUP

Preparation Time: 10 minutes
Cooking time: 20 minutes
Servings: 2

Ingredients:

- 2 tablespoons coconut oil
- 2 garlic cloves, minced
- 1 inch fresh ginger root, peeled and minced
- 1 onion, sliced
- 6 cremini mushrooms, sliced
- 1 red bell pepper, chopped
- 1 green bell pepper, chopped
- 3 baby red potatoes, quartered
- 2 tablespoons curry powder
- 1 tablespoon red curry paste (optional)
- 2 tablespoons tamari (gluten-free soy sauce)
- 4 cups vegetable broth or bone broth for a non-vegan variation (homemade, here, or store-bought organic)
- 1 (16-ounce) can coconut milk
- Sea salt
- Freshly ground black pepper
- 5 fresh basil leaves, cut into thin ribbons

Directions:

1. In a large pot over medium heat, melt the coconut oil. Add the garlic, ginger, and onions, and sauté until the onion is translucent, 3 to 4 minutes.
2. Add the mushrooms, red and green peppers, potatoes, curry powder, curry paste, and tamari, and stir until well combined.
3. Add the broth and coconut milk. Bring to a simmer for 15 minutes, or until the potatoes can be pierced easily with a fork.
4. Salt and pepper to taste. Ladle into 2 bowls, top with the basil, and serve.

Nutrition: *Calories: 915; Total fat: 69g; Saturated fat: 60g; Sodium: 1,068mg; Carbohydrates: 72g; Fiber: 17g; Protein: 16g*

DEVILED EGG SALAD

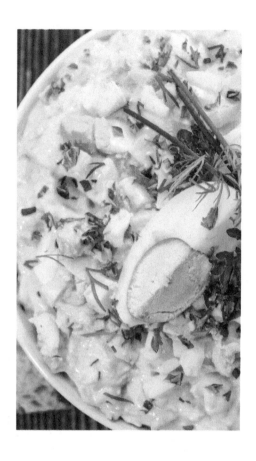

Preparation Time: 15 minutes
Servings: 3 to 4

Ingredients:

- 6 large hard-boiled eggs, peeled, cooled, and roughly chopped
- ¼ cup thinly sliced scallions, white and green parts
- ½ cup minced celery
- 1 red bell pepper, minced
- 1 tablespoon Dijon mustard
- ¼ cup Homemade Almond Mayo
- ½ teaspoon paprika, plus more for garnish
- Sea salt
- Freshly ground black pepper

Directions:

1. In a large bowl, combine the chopped eggs, scallions, celery, bell pepper, mustard, Homemade Almond Mayo, and paprika. Season with salt and pepper.
2. Mix well, adding more mayo if needed.
3. Sprinkle with a little extra paprika on top and serve.

Nutrition: *Calories: 225; Total fat: 16g; Saturated fat: 4g; Sodium: 237mg; Carbohydrates: 10g; Fiber: 1g; Protein: 12g*

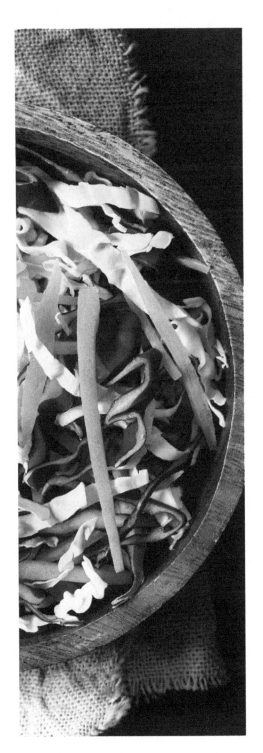

CARROT AND BEET COLESLAW

Preparation Time: 10 minutes
Servings: 2

Ingredients:
- 3 large carrots, peeled and shredded (you can use a food processor or cheese grater)
- 2 large beets, peeled and shredded
- 1 large green apple, cored and shredded
- 1 tablespoon fresh dill, minced
- 1 tablespoon freshly squeezed lemon juice
- ¼ cup plain Greek yogurt
- ¼ cup toasted pumpkin seeds

Directions:
1. In a large salad bowl, combine the carrots, beets, apple, dill, lemon juice, yogurt, and pumpkin seeds. Mix well and serve.

Nutrition: *Calories: 265; Total fat: 9g; Saturated fat: 2g; Sodium: 173mg; Carbohydrates: 41g; Fiber: 8g; Protein: 10g*

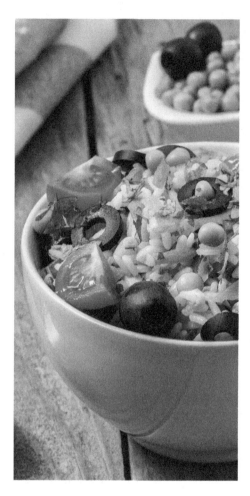

HEARTY WINTER SALAD WITH FORBIDDEN RICE

Preparation Time: 20 minutes
Cooking time: 15 minutes
Servings: 4

Ingredients:

- 2 yams, peeled and cut into cubes
- 2 tablespoons coconut oil or ghee
- Sea salt
- Freshly ground black pepper
- 1 ripe avocado, pitted and cut into cubes
- ½ cup dried cranberries
- ¼ cup sliced almonds
- ¼ cup toasted pumpkin seeds
- 1 bag mixed greens
- 1 cup forbidden or wild rice, cooked
- ¼ cup homemade Green Goddess Dressing

Directions:

1. Preheat the oven to 420°F.
2. On a cookie sheet, toss the chopped yams with the oil and spread evenly. Sprinkle with salt and pepper.
3. Roast for 15 minutes, or until tender and golden. Set aside to cool.
4. Once the yams have cooled, combine them in a large bowl with the avocado, cranberries, almonds, pumpkin seeds, greens, and rice. Toss with Green Goddess Dressing, mix well, and serve.

Nutrition: *Calories: 392; Total fat: 21g; Saturated fat: 8g; Sodium: 31mg; Carbohydrates: 48g; Fiber: 9g; Protein: 8g*

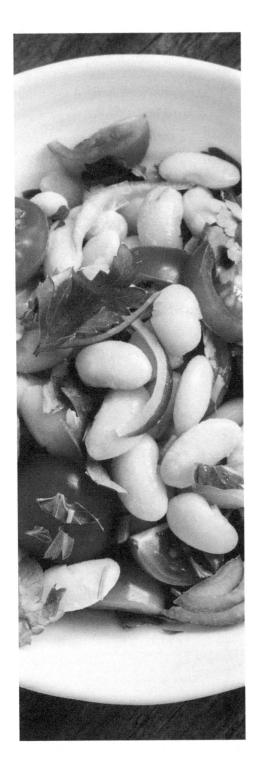

ROASTED VEGETABLE AND WHITE BEAN SALAD

Preparation Time: 15 minutes
Cooking time: 10 minutes
Servings: 4

Ingredients:

FOR THE SALAD

- 1 red bell pepper, cored and chopped into cubes
- 1 yellow bell pepper, cored and chopped into cubes
- 1 green bell pepper, cored and chopped into cubes
- 1 yam, peeled and cut into small cubes
- 1 cup cremini mushrooms, quartered
- 1 zucchini, cut into half moons
- ½ cup avocado oil
- Sea salt
- Freshly ground black pepper
- 1 (16-ounce) can white beans, rinsed
- 1 cup fresh, baby spinach

FOR THE DRESSING

- ¼ cup olive oil
- ¼ cup apple cider vinegar (I use Bragg's)
- 1 teaspoon nutritional yeast flakes
- Sea salt
- Freshly ground black pepper

Directions:

1. Preheat the oven to 400°F.
2. On a large sheet pan, toss the bell peppers, yams, mushrooms, and zucchini with the avocado oil, and liberally sprinkle with salt and pepper.
3. Roast for 10 to 12 minutes, until everything is golden and tender.
4. Meanwhile, in a small bowl, make the dressing by mixing together the olive oil, apple cider vinegar, and nutritional yeast flakes. Season with salt and pepper to taste.
5. In a large bowl, mix the warm, roasted vegetables, beans, and dressing.
6. Lay the fresh baby spinach on the bottom of a large serving bowl, and serve the roasted vegetables on top of the spinach.

Nutrition: *Calories: 392; Total fat: 17g; Saturated fat: 3g; Sodium: 237mg; Carbohydrates: 51g; Fiber: 15g; Protein: 12g*

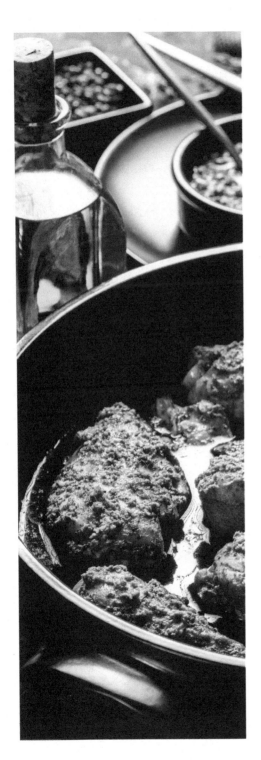

PUMPKIN SEED PESTO CHICKEN AND ARUGULA SANDWICH

Preparation Time: 10 minutes
Cooking time: 35 minutes
Servings: 2

Ingredients:
- 2 chicken breasts
- 1 tablespoon avocado oil
- ¼ teaspoon sea salt, plus more for seasoning
- Freshly ground black pepper
- 3 garlic cloves, peeled and minced
- 1 cup fresh basil leaves, roughly chopped
- 1 cup fresh parsley, roughly chopped
- ½ cup pumpkin seeds
- ¼ teaspoon salt
- ¼ cup olive oil
- 4 slices gluten-free bread, toasted
- 1 cup arugula

Directions:

1. Preheat the oven to 375ºF.
2. Place the chicken breasts in a small baking dish. Drizzle with the avocado oil, and sprinkle with salt and pepper. Roast for 35 minutes, or until brown on top and cooked through. Set aside.
3. In a blender or food processor, combine the garlic, basil, parsley, pumpkin seeds, salt, and olive oil. Blend well, adding more oil if necessary to get a saucy, smooth, spreadable consistency.
4. Spread the pesto liberally on all 4 slices of bread, top with arugula and chicken before closing the sandwich, and serve.

Nutrition: *Calories: 424; Total fat: 29g; Saturated fat: 6g; Sodium: 508mg; Carbohydrates: 25g; Fiber: 2g; Protein: 20g*

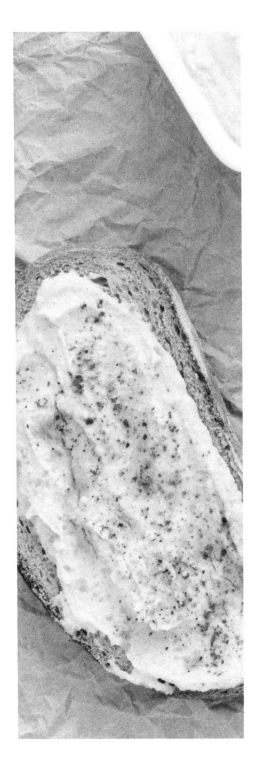

HUMMUS VEGETABLE SANDWICH

Preparation Time: 25 minutes
Cooking time: 5 minutes
Servings: 2

Ingredients:

- 1 (16-ounce) can chickpeas, drained, liquid reserved
- 2 tablespoons olive oil
- 3 garlic cloves, minced
- ½ teaspoon salt
- ¼ teaspoon freshly ground black pepper
- 3 tablespoons tahini (sesame seed paste)
- 2 teaspoons freshly squeezed lemon juice
- ¼ teaspoon ground cumin
- ¼ teaspoon paprika
- 4 slices gluten-free bread
- 1 Persian cucumber, sliced into thin discs
- 1 carrot, sliced into thin discs
- 1 cup broccoli sprouts

Instructions:

1. In a food processor or blender, combine the chickpeas, olive oil, garlic, salt, pepper, tahini, lemon juice, cumin, and paprika. While blending, slowly add 1 tablespoon of the reserved chickpea liquid to bring the hummus to a smooth consistency. Set aside.
2. Toast the bread, then liberally spread the hummus on all 4 slices.
3. Arrange the cucumber and carrot discs on the hummus, then add the broccoli sprouts.
4. Sprinkle with a bit of extra salt and paprika if desired, before closing the sandwiches and slicing to serve.

Nutrition: *Calories: 720; Total fat: 33g; Saturated fat: 7g; Sodium: 1,476mg; Carbohydrates: 93g; Fiber: 17g; Protein: 21g*

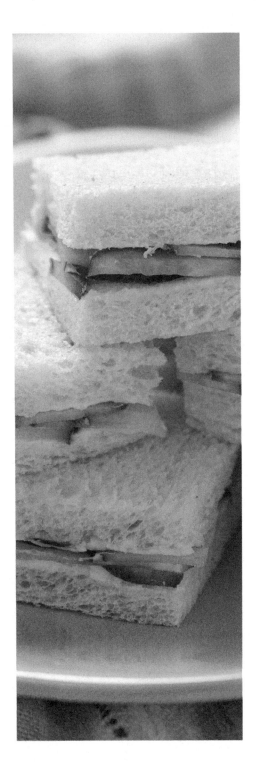

GREEN GODDESS CUCUMBER TEA SANDWICHES

Preparation Time: 15 minutes
Servings: 2

Ingredients:

- 1 ripe avocado, pitted
- 2 tablespoons freshly squeezed lemon juice
- 1 teaspoon minced fresh dill
- 1 garlic clove, peeled and minced
- Sea salt
- ½ cup homemade Green Goddess Dressing
- 2 Persian cucumbers, sliced into discs
- 4 slices gluten-free bread

Directions:

1. Scoop the avocado flesh into a small bowl, and mash with a spoon until creamy.
2. Stir in the lemon juice, dill, garlic, and salt to taste.
3. In another small bowl, combine the Green Goddess Dressing with the cucumbers.
4. Spread some avocado mixture on each slice of bread, then arrange your dressed cucumber discs neatly atop before closing up the sandwiches. I like to use 2 layers of cucumbers for maximum crunch.
5. Slice into quarters, and serve with a cup of digestive tea. Keep that pinky up!

Nutrition: *Calories: 357; Total fat: 18g; Saturated fat: 5g; Sodium: 781mg; Carbohydrates: 46g; Fiber: 9g; Protein: 8g*

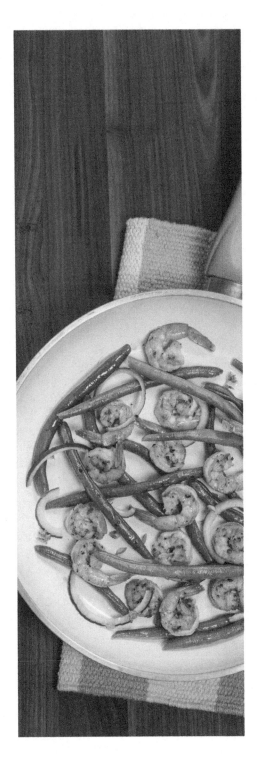

SHRIMP WITH BEANS

Preparation Time: 10 minutes
Cooking time: 10 minutes
Servings: 4

Ingredients:

- 1 Lb. shrimp, peeled and deveined
- 2 Tbsp. soy sauce
- ½ Lb. green beans, washed and trimmed
- 2 Tbsp. olive oil
- Salt

Directions:

1. Heat oil in a pan.
2. Add beans to the pan and sauté for 5-6 minutes or until tender.
3. Remove pan from heat and set aside.
4. Add shrimp in the same pan and cook for 2-3 minutes each side.
5. Return beans to the pan along with soy sauce. Stir well and cook until shrimp is done.
6. Season with salt and serve.

Nutrition: *Calories: 217, Total Fat: 9g, Saturated Fat: 1.6g, Protein: 27.4g, Carbs: 6.4g, Fiber: 2g, Sugar: 0.9g*

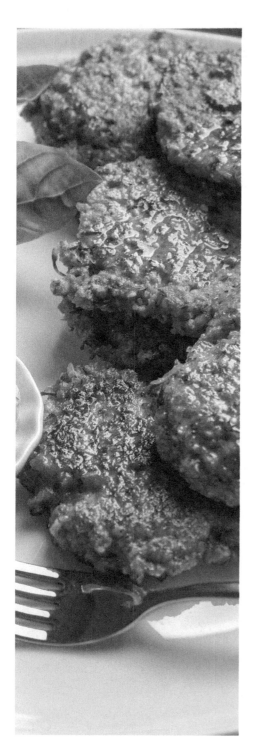

BROCCOLI FRITTERS

Preparation Time: 10 minutes
Cooking time: 15 minutes
Servings: 4

Ingredients:

- 3 cups broccoli florets
- 1/3 cup parmesan cheese, grated
- ½ cup flour, gluten-free
- 1 large egg, lightly beaten
- 2 Tbsp. olive oil
- Pepper
- Salt

Directions:

1. Steam broccoli florets until tender. Let it cool completely and chop.
2. In a bowl, add egg, cheese, flour, pepper, and salt. Mix well.
3. Add chopped broccoli into the egg mixture and mix well. If the mixture is too dry, then add a tablespoon of water.
4. Heat the olive oil in a pan over medium heat.
5. Make patties from the mixture and cook on the hot pan for 3 minutes each side.
6. Serve and enjoy.

Nutrition: *Calories: 208, Total Fat: 11.6g, Saturated Fat: 3.4g, Protein: 9.1g, Carbs: 16.6g, Fiber: 2.2g, Sugar: 1.3g*

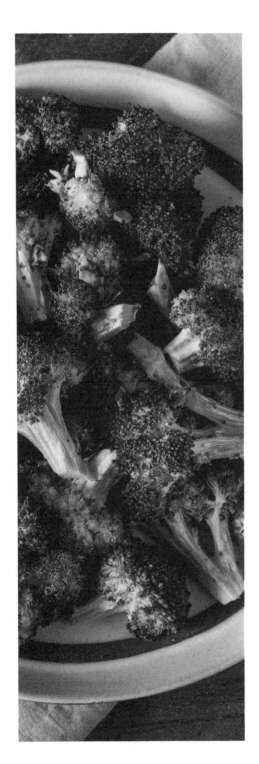

ROASTED BROCCOLI

Preparation Time: 10 minutes
Cooking time: 15 minutes
Servings: 8

Ingredients:

- 8 cups broccoli florets
- ½ Tsp. Red chili flakes
- 2 Tbsp. soy sauce
- ¼ cup olive oil

Directions:

1. Preheat the oven to 425 F
2. Spray a baking tray w/ cooking spray and set aside.
3. Add all of the ingredients to the large mixing bowl and toss well—transfer broccoli mixture on a prepared baking tray.
4. Roast in preheated oven for 15 minutes.
5. Serve and enjoy.

Nutrition: *Calories: 87, Total Fat: 6.6g, Saturated Fat: 0.9g, Protein: 2.8g,Carbs: 6.3g, Fiber: 2.4g,*

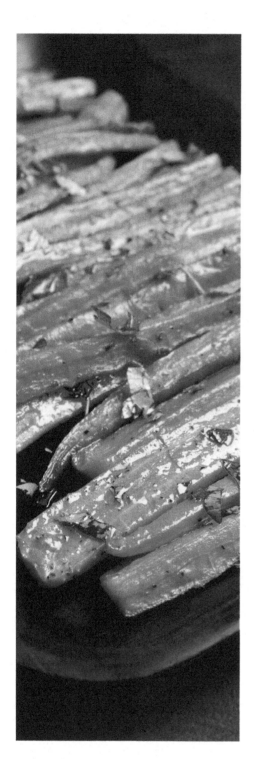

ROASTED MAPLE CARROTS

Preparation Time: 10 minutes
Cooking time: 25 minutes
Servings: 3

Ingredients:

- 1 Lb. baby carrots
- 2 Tsp. Fresh parsley, chopped
- 1 Tbsp. Dijon mustard
- 2 Tbsp. butter, melted
- 3 Tbsp. maple syrup
- Pepper
- Salt

Directions:

1. Preheat the oven to 400 o F
2. In a large bowl, toss carrots with Dijon mustard, maple syrup, butter, pepper, and salt.
3. Transfer carrots to baking tray and spread evenly.
4. Roast carrots in preheated oven for 25-30 minutes.
5. Serve and enjoy.

Nutrition: *Calories: 177, Total Fat: 8.1g, Saturated Fat: 4.9g, Protein: 1.3g,Carbs: 26.2g, Fiber: 4.6g, Sugar: 19.2g*

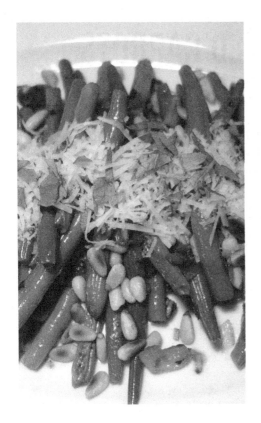

SWEET & TANGY GREEN BEANS

Preparation Time: 10 minutes
Cooking time: 15 minutes
Servings: 6

Ingredients:
- 1 ½ Lb. green beans, trimmed
- 1 Tbsp. maple syrup
- 2 Tbsp. Dijon mustard
- 2 Tbsp. rice wine vinegar
- ¼ cup olive oil
- ½ cup pecans, chopped
- Pepper
- Salt

Directions:
1. Preheat the oven to 400 o F
2. Place pecans on baking tray and toast in preheated oven for 5-8 minutes.
3. Remove from the oven and let it cool.
4. Boil a water in a large pot over high heat.
5. Add green beans in boiling water and cook for 4-5 minutes or until tender. Drain beans well and place in a large bowl.
6. Whisk together oil, maple syrup, mustard, and vinegar in a bowl.
7. Season beans with pepper and salt. Pour oil mixture over green beans.
8. Add pecans and toss well.
9. Serve and enjoy.

Nutrition: *Calories: 139, Total Fat: 10.4g, Saturated Fat: 1.4g, Protein: 2.5g, Carbs: 10.9g, Fiber: 4.3g, Sugar: 3.7g*

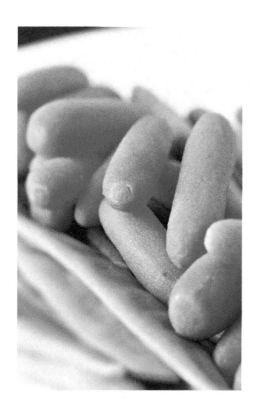

SAUTÉED CARROTS AND BEANS

Preparation Time: 10 minutes
Cooking time: 10 minutes
Servings: 2

Ingredients:
- 2 cups green beans, trimmed
- 1 Tbsp. fresh lemon juice
- 2 Tbsp. butter
- 1 cup baby carrots, halved lengthwise
- 1 Tbsp. olive oil
- Pepper
- Salt

Directions:
1. Heat olive oil in a large pan.
2. Add carrots to the pan & cook for a minute.
3. Add green beans and cook until beans are just tender, season with pepper and salt.
4. Once vegetables are cooked, then remove from pan and place on a plate.
5. Turn heat to medium-low and add butter in the same pan. Once butter is melted, then add lemon juice and stir well.
6. Return vegetables to the pan and toss well to coat.
7. Serve and enjoy.

Nutrition: *Calories: 233, Total Fat: 18.7g, Saturated Fat: 8.4g, Protein: 2.2g, Carbs: 16g, Fiber: 6.8g, Sugar: 6.7g*

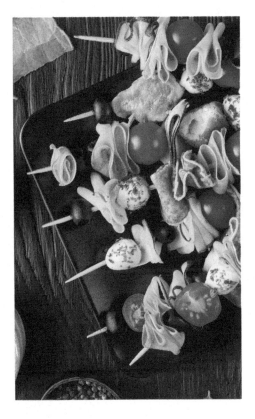

ANTIPASTO ON A STICK

Preparation Time: 5 minutes
Cooking time: 0 minutes
Servings: 1

Ingredients:
- 1 small jar pepperoncini
- 1 small jar pitted Kalamata olives
- Fresh mozzarella balls, small, 2 for each skewer
- Thinly sliced ham or Canadian bacon
- Basil leaves or spinach leaves
- Grape tomatoes
- Skewers about 6 inches long

Directions:
1. Cut the pepperoncini in half so that it will fit evenly on the skewer.
2. Fold the ham into quarters to fit on the skewer.
3. Layer the ingredients on the skewer, placing 2 mozzarella balls, 2 slices of ham, 1 whole pepperoncino, and 2 grape tomatoes on each skewer. Add olives between the Ingredients as you desire.
4. Nutrition Information is based on 5 olives per skewer.
5. Serve on a platter with spinach leaves scattered around for a beautiful presentation.

Nutrition: *Calories: 263 Fat: 17g Carbs: 8 g Protein: 22 g*

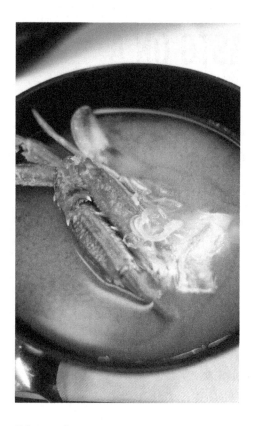

CRAB AND MISO SOUP

Servings: 4

Ingredients:

- 2 x 250g pots Instant Brown
- Medium Grain Rice in 90 seconds
- 2 bunches broccoli, stems sliced
- 2 corn cobs
- 1/3 cup white miso paste
- 1/4 cup tahini
- 200g fresh crab meat, cooked
- 1/3 cup chopped chives
- 2 teaspoons black sesame seeds, toasted

Directions:

1. Cook rice following the package directions.
2. Add 6 cups of water in a large saucepan. Bring the water to boil over high heat. Add the broccoli and cook for 1 min. Meanwhile, cut corn kernels from the fresh cobs.
3. Add to the pan with rice and cook for 1 minute. Remove from heat.
4. Add miso paste and tahini and stir until well combined—divide between 4 serving bowls.
5. Add the crab and sprinkle with chives and sesame seeds.

Nutrition: *Calories: 514.50 Fat: 15g –Carbs: 82.60g Protein: 22.50g*

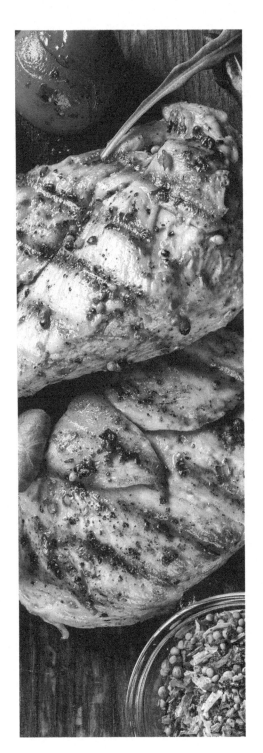

MEXICAN LIME CHICKEN

Servings: 4

Ingredients:

- 1 Lb. boneless, and skinless chicken breasts, pounded to an even thickness
- 1/4 cup fresh lime juice
- 2 tablespoons olive oil
- 1/2 teaspoon ancho chili powder
- 1/2 teaspoon salt
- 1/4 teaspoon fresh ground black pepper

Directions:

1. Make a marinade of lime juice, ancho chili powder, salt, and pepper. Pour this into a sealable plastic bag or bowl and place the chicken breasts inside, poking them first with a fork so they will absorb more marinade. Refrigerate for two hours, turning the chicken over every 30 minutes to ensure it is coated evenly.
2. Drain the chicken and grill over medium until the chicken is done.

Nutrition: *Calories: 204 Fat: 10 g Carbs: 1 g Protein: 26g*

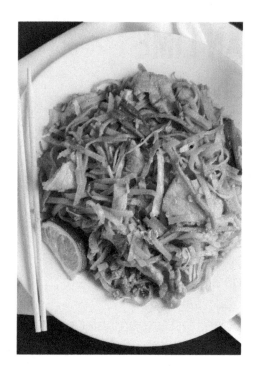

PAD THAI NOODLES

Servings: 4

Ingredients:

- 250g rice stick noodles
- 2 tablespoons Rice Oil
- 2 eggs, scrambled a bit · 1/3 cup pad Thai paste
- 250g firm tofu, chopped into fine pieces
- 100g beansprouts end trimmed
- 2 tablespoons peanuts, chopped coarsely
- Lime wedges, for garnish

Directions:

1. Add the rice noodles in a heatproof bowl. Cover w/ boiling hot water. Stand for 10 minutes until softened. Drain the noodles in a colander. Set the noodles aside.
2. Heat 1 Tsp. Of oil in a large frying pan. Add egg and fry softly enough that the white is set. Cook for 2 minutes and remove to a plate. Roughly chop the egg.
3. Heat the remaining oil in the pan. Add the Thai paste and tofu. Stir together in the oil for 1 minute or until fragrant. Add the rice noodles. Cook, stirring, for 1 minute or until the noodles are warmed. Remove from heat.
4. Divide the noodle mixture between the serving bowls. Place the beansprouts on top, then the pieces of egg, then the peanuts. Squirt a spritz of lime juice into the noodles and serve with decorative lime pieces.

Nutrition: *Calories: 380 Fat: 21g Carbs: 28g Protein: 16 g*

PARMESAN COATED WINGS

Servings: 2

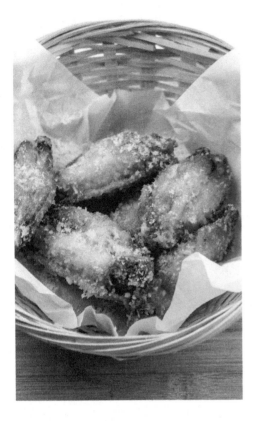

Ingredients:

- 24 chicken wings
- Olive oil cooking spray
- 1 tablespoon garlic-flavored olive oil
- 3 tablespoons butter
- 1/4 teaspoon salt
- 1/4 teaspoon ground black pepper
- 1/2 cup finely shredded
- Parmesan cheese
- Chopped fresh parsley

Directions:

1. Preheat oven to 370° F. Line a large baking sheet with aluminum foil, shiny side up, and spritz with olive oil cooking spray. Place the wings on the prepared sheet and season with salt and pepper. Bake for 1 hour, or until golden brown.
2. In a small saucepan, heat olive oil. Add butter and melt to combine with the oil. Stir in salt and pepper.
3. Arrange wings on a serving plate and drizzle with the butter and oil mixture. Sprinkle with Parmesan cheese and chopped parsley and serve.

Nutrition: *Calories: 142 Fat: 11g Carbs: 0g Protein: 11g*

PINA COLADA BITES

Servings: 4

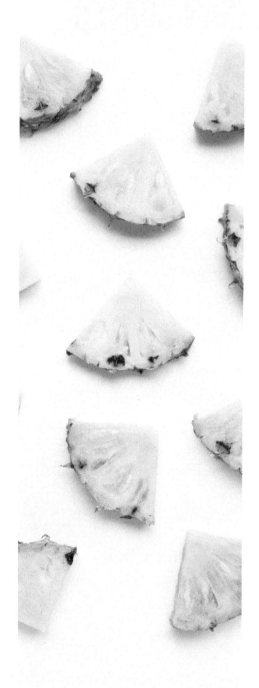

Ingredients:
- 1.3kg pineapple
- 1 1/2 cups caster sugar
- 1 cup of water
- 1 tablespoon of liquid glucose
- 2 teaspoons Coconut extract

Directions:
1. Cut the pineapple slices into smaller bits.
2. Combine the sugars and water into a saucepan, stirring until all the sugars are melted. Bring the liquid to a simmer. Add the pineapple and 2 teaspoons coconut extract. Slowly continue to simmer for 40 minutes or until the pineapple is opaque.
3. Use a slotted spoon to transfer to a rack placed over a baking tray lined with baking paper.
4. Preheat oven to 225F. Bake for 1 1/4 hours, to dry the pineapple. Allow the pineapple to cool. Store in an airtight container at room temperature or refrigerate if the atmosphere is humid.

Nutrition: *Calories: 460Fat: 4g Carbs: 107g Protein: 1.8 g*

SAVORY CHICKEN AND RICE MUFFINS

Servings: 8

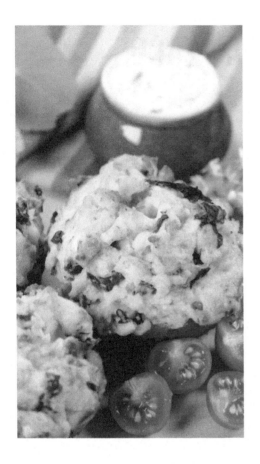

Ingredients:

- 2/3 cup Basmati Rice
- 250g skinless smoked chicken breast, chopped finely
- 2/3 cup dried tomatoes, coarsely chopped
- 1 1/3 cups grated fresh mozzarella cheese
- 3 green onions, thinly sliced, the green tops only
- 1/4 cup basil leaves, chopped finely
- 3 eggs, lightly beaten

Directions:

1. Preheat oven to 400F. Grease Texas-sized muffin tin. Line the muffin tin with liners.
2. Cook the basmati rice as the package suggests. Rinse the rice and let cool.
3. Place all ingredients into a bowl, with the exception of 1/3 cups of the mozzarella cheese.
4. Spoon the mixture of chicken and rice into the prepared muffin pan. Sprinkle with remaining cheese. Bake for 15 to 20 mins. or until the muffins are firm & light golden in color. Stand in pan for 5 minutes. Dump the muffins onto a plate and allow it to cool. Store in an airtight container. Refrigerate until ready to serve. Enjoy for breakfast or as a light tea snack.

Nutrition: *Calories: 229 Fat: 8 g Carbs: 18g Protein: 20g*

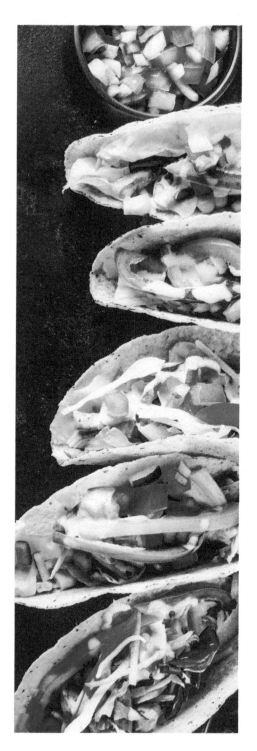

TUESDAY TACOS

Servings: 4

Ingredients:

- 1 jalapeno chilies (diced) optional
- 1 handful chives (diced)
- 2 red pepper (green and, diced)
- 2 Lbs. ground chicken (or turkey)
- 1 can diced tomatoes (with or without chilies)
- 2 tbsps. Cumin
- 2 tbsps. Paprika
- 1 tbsp. cayenne pepper
- 1 tbsp. oregano

Directions:

1. Start with placing the chives, bell pepper pieces, and the ground chicken, with a tablespoon of olive into a skillet and beginning to fry.
2. Fry the meat and the peppers until the meat is no longer pink, the meat is crumbled, and the peppers are soft.
3. Sprinkle spices into your meat and mix, occasionally tasting for flavor. When the meat has the desired flavor, add the can of diced tomatoes and serve.

Nutrition: *Calories: 390 Fat: 20 g Carbs: 11g Protein: 41g*

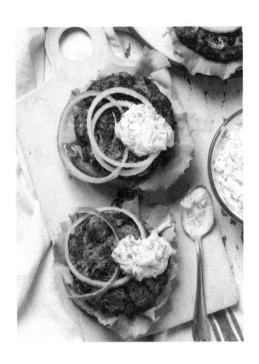

TURKEY BURGERS WITH SPINACH AND FETA

Servings: 4

Ingredients:
- 1 Lb. ground turkey
- 1 egg beaten
- 1 cup crumbled feta cheese
- 3 cups frozen spinach, defrosted
- Spices of your choice: paprika, oregano, cayenne pepper, salt, pepper
- Olive oil

Directions:
1. Place your ingredients into a bowl and mix together.
2. Scoop one Pattie together and press until firm.
3. Place gently into the cooking oil in a skillet on medium.
4. Place each Pattie into the pan in this manner.
5. Let the patties cook for 7 minutes on one side,
6. then gently turn so the patties will stay firm and shaped.
7. Flip the patties & cook for another 6 or 7 minutes.
8. Serve

Nutrition: *Calories: 360 Fat: 24 g Carbs: 9g Protein: 28g*

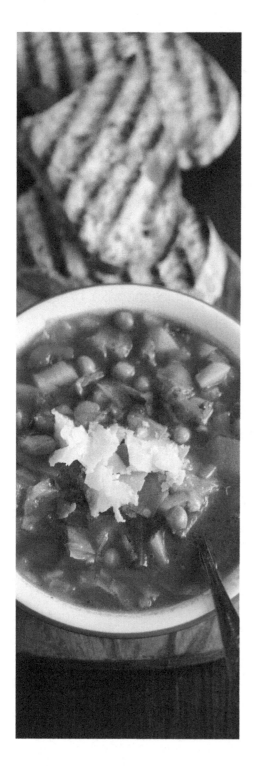

MINESTRONE

Preparation Time: 10 minutes
Cooking time: 40 minutes
Servings: 4

Ingredients:

- 65 grams middle bacon
- 80 grams leek
- 75 grams shell pasta, gluten-free
- 240 grams carrots, diced
- 12 grams fresh basil, chopped
- 160 grams potato, diced
- 310 milliliters boiling water
- 50 grams celery, sliced
- 160 grams zucchini, diced
- 2 tablespoons garlic-infused oil
- 400 grams canned plain tomatoes, chopped
- 60 grams spinach, sliced
- 3 tablespoons parmesan cheese
- Olive oil
- Salt and pepper
- 500 milliliters vegetable stock
- 168 grams canned chickpeas, rinsed and drained

Directions:

1. Remove the white stem of the leeks.
2. Chop the green tips finely and set aside.
3. Slice the bacon into small pieces after removing the rind.
4. Over medium heat, saute carrots, potato, leeks, bacon and celery in a large saucepan using garlic-infused oil for about 20 minutes.
5. Add tomatoes, boiling water, chickpeas, vegetable stock, spinach and zucchini into the pan. T
6. urn down the heat to medium-low and let it simmer. After 10 minutes, put the pasta and basil in the pan.
7. Allow the pasta to cook in the soup. Sprinkle salt and pepper to taste.
8. Adjust the soup's consistency by adding water, if desired. Serve with parmesan cheese, baby basil leaves and an extra drizzle of garlic-infused oil.

Nutrition: *Calories: 386 Total Fat: 17 g Saturated Fat: 0 g Cholesterol: 0 mg Sodium: mg Total Carbs: 50.4 g Fiber: 10.6 g Sugar: 11.8 g Protein: 11.9 g*

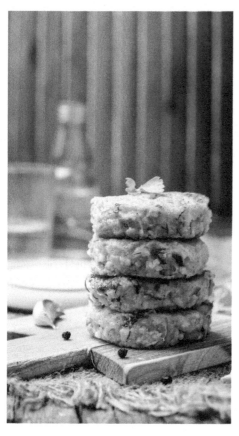

CHEESY CHICKEN FRITTERS

Preparation Time: 10 minutes
Cooking time: 20 minutes
Servings: 4

Ingredients:

- 500 grams chicken, ground
- 84 grams mozzarella cheese, grated
- ¼ teaspoon salt
- 2 large eggs
- 2 teaspoons chives, dried
- 60 milliliters mayonnaise
- 2 tablespoons fresh basil, chopped
- 35 grams plain flour, gluten-free
- Olive oil
- Black pepper

Directions:

1. Mix all of the ingredients thoroughly in a large bowl.
2. Season with salt and pepper.
3. Place a large frying pan with olive oil over medium heat.
4. Scoop about ¼ cup of the chicken mixture and place it in the pan.
5. Flatten the mixture slightly using a spatula and let it cook for about 4 minutes on each side.
6. Line a plate with paper towel.
7. Once cooked thoroughly, transfer the fritters into the plate to remove excess oil.
8. Repeat the process for the remaining chicken mixture.

Nutrition: *Calories: 415 Total Fat: 26.8 g Saturated Fat: 0 g Cholesterol: 0 mg Sodium: 0 mg Total Carbs: 11.4 g Fiber: 0.4 g Sugar: 1.7 g Protein: 31.3 g*

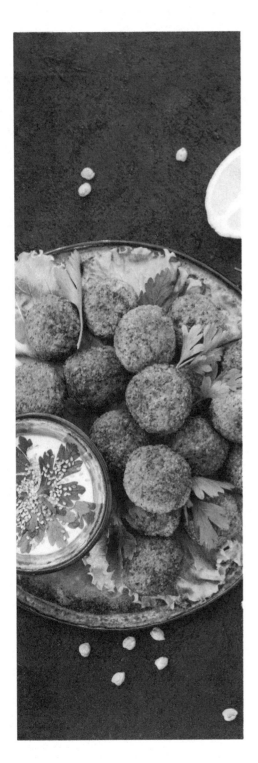

CRISPY FALAFEL

Preparation Time: 10 minutes
Cooking time: 25 minutes
Servings: 5

Ingredients:

- 120 grams carrots, grated and peeled
- 2 tablespoons olive oil
- 5 tablespoons plain flour, gluten-free
- ¾ teaspoon cumin, ground
- 25 grams fresh parsley, chopped
- 2 teaspoons paprika
- 80 grams leek
- 2 tablespoons garlic-infused oil
- Zest and juice of 1 large lime
- Salt and pepper
- 182 grams microwavable brown rice, pre-cooked
- 168 grams canned chickpeas, rinsed and drained

Directions:

1. Set the oven to 380°F. Prepare a roasting tray lined with baking paper.
2. Remove the white stems of the leek and chop the green tips roughly. Except for the plain flour, blend all of the ingredients using a food processor.
3. Once the mixture becomes a smooth paste, add the plain flour and mix well. Use 1 tablespoon of olive oil to grease the baking paper. Form small falafel patties using a tablespoon and place them on the roasting tray. Make sure to allocate enough space between each patty.
4. Coat the top of the patties with olive oil. Place the tray in the oven and cook for about 12 minutes on each side.

Nutrition: *Calories: 187 Total Fat: 7.1 g Saturated Fat: 0 g Cholesterol: 0 mg Sodium: 0 mg Total Carbs: 27.7 g Fiber: 4.5 g Sugar: 3.6 g Protein: 4.4 g*

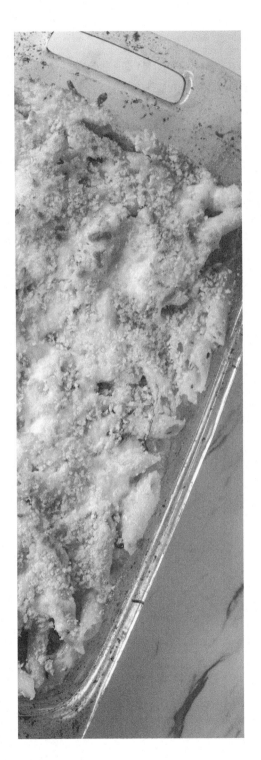

CHICKEN ALFREDO PASTA BAKE

Preparation Time: 10 minutes
Cooking time: 50 minutes
Servings: 4

Ingredients:

- 450 grams chicken breast
- 3 tablespoons fresh sage, chopped
- 5 tablespoons butter
- 114 grams cheddar cheese, grated
- ¼ cup plain flour, gluten-free
- 20 grams green onions
- 750 milliliters rice milk
- 180 grams broccoli florets
- 3 tablespoons parmesan cheese, grated
- 120 grams baby spinach, chopped
- ½ teaspoon basil, dried
- 240 grams pasta, gluten-free
- Salt and pepper
- Olive oil

Directions:

1. Heat the oven to 360°F. Apply olive oil on a large oven dish to grease it. Slice the chicken breast fillet into small pieces. Sear the chicken using olive oil in a large frying pan over medium-high heat.

2. Once the meat is golden brown, remove it from the flame and set aside for later.

3. Remove the white stems of the green onions and chop the green tips finely. Place the spinach leaves in a hot pan until slightly wilted. Remove from heat and place it on one side for later use. Over medium heat, melt the butter in a medium-sized saucepan.

4. Add plain flour into the saucepan and stir continuously for a minute while cooking. Once slightly frothy, add ½ cup of milk into the saucepan and stir until smooth. P

5. our 1 cup of milk at a time into the mixture while stirring continuously. Season to taste. Add parmesan cheese, basil and 57 grams of cheddar cheese into the sauce.

6. Give the mixture an occasional stir until it gained a thick consistency. Prepare a large saucepan of boiling water and cook the pasta. After 5 minutes, drain the pasta and drizzle with olive oil.

7. Add Alfredo sauce, broccoli, chicken and spinach into the pasta and mix well. Transfer everything to the greased oven dish and sprinkle the remaining cheese on top.

8. Let it cook in the oven for 10 minutes without cover. Place the pasta bake in an oven grill and cook for another 3 minutes. Garnish with sage.

Nutrition: *Calories: 743 Total Fat: 29.9 g Saturated Fat: 0 g Cholesterol: 0 mg Sodium: 0 mg Total Carbs: 78.8 g Fiber: 10 g Sugar: 11.4 g Protein: 41 g*

CHAPTER FIVE:

Dinners

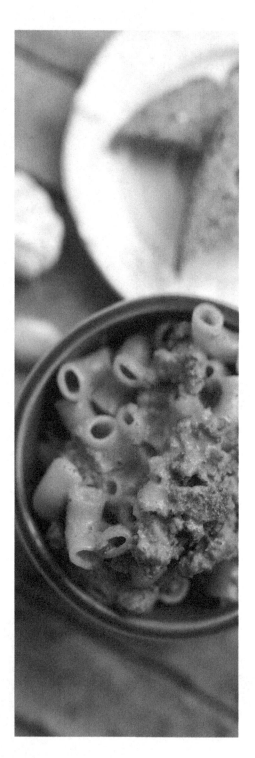

CHEESEBURGER MACARONI

Preparation Time: 10 minutes
Cooking time: 25 minutes
Servings: 4

Ingredients:

- 1 Lb. ground beef
- 1 cup cheddar cheese, shredded
- 1 Tsp. Chili powder
- 1 ½ Tbsp. prepared mustard
- ¼ cup ketchup
- ½ cup of water
- 14.5 Oz. can tomatoes, diced
- 2 scallions, sliced green part only
- 3 bacon slices, chopped
- 8 Oz. elbow pasta, gluten-free
- ¼ Tsp. Pepper
- ½ Tsp. Salt

Directions:

1. Cook macaroni according to packet instructions. Drain well and set aside.
2. Heat large pan over medium heat. Add bacon slices to the pan and sauté until crispy.
3. Add scallions and beef to the pan and sauté until meat is no longer pink.
4. Transfer meat to a paper towel-lined dish to drain grease.
5. Add meat, tomatoes, chili powder, mustard, ketchup, water, pepper, and salt into the same pan. Bring to simmer for 5 minutes.
6. Add cheese and cooked macaroni to the pan and cook until cheese is melted about 5 minutes.
7. Serve and enjoy.

Nutrition: *Calories: 659; Total Fat: 24.3g; Saturated Fat: 11.1g; Protein: 55.5g; Carbs: 52.4g; Fiber: 7.5g; Sugar: 8.3g*

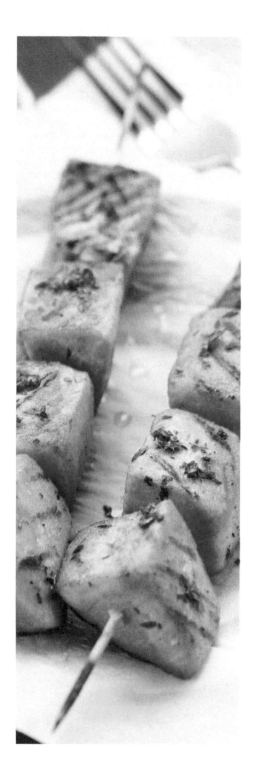

SALMON SKEWERS

Preparation Time: 10 minutes
Cooking time: 10 minutes
Servings: 4

Ingredients:

- 1 Lb. salmon fillets, cut into 1-inch cubes
- 2 Tbsp. soy sauce
- 1 Tbsp. sesame seeds, toasted
- 1 ½ Tbsp. maple syrup
- 1 Tsp. Ginger, crushed
- 1 lime juice
- 1 lime zest
- 2 Tsp. Olive oil

Directions:

1. In a bowl, mix together olive oil, soy sauce, lime zest, lime juice, maple syrup, and ginger.
2. Add salmon and stir to coat. Set aside for 10 minutes.
3. Slide marinated salmon pieces onto soaked wooden skewers and grill for 8-10 minutes or until cooked.
4. Sprinkle salmon skewers w/ sesame seeds and serve.

Nutrition: *Calories:211; Total Fat: 10.5g; Saturated Fat: 1.5g; Protein: 23g;Carbs: 7.4g; Fiber: 0.4g; Sugar: 4.8g*

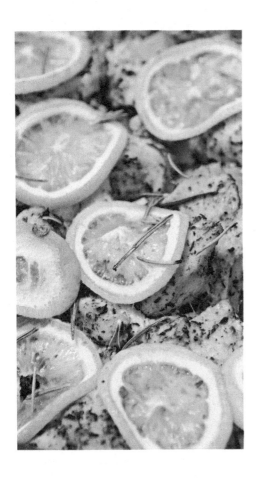

LEMON CHICKEN

Preparation Time: 10 minutes
Cooking time: 4 hours
Servings: 4

Ingredients:
- 20 Oz. chicken breasts, skinless, boneless, and cut into pieces
- ¾ cup chicken broth,
- ½ cup fresh lemon juice
- 1/8 Tsp. Dried thyme
- ¼ Tsp. Dried basil
- ½ Tsp. Dried oregano
- 1 Tsp. Dried parsley
- 2 Tbsp. olive oil
- 2 Tbsp. butter
- 3 Tbsp. rice flour
- 1 Tsp. Salt

Directions:
1. In a bowl, toss chicken with rice flour.
2. Heat the butter, and olive oil in a pan over medium-high heat.
3. Add chicken to the pan and cook until brown.
4. Transfer chicken to the slow cooker. Add remaining ingredients on top of chicken.
5. Cover slow cooker w/ lid and cook on low for 4 hours.
6. Serve and enjoy.

Nutrition: *Calories: 423; Total Fat: 23.9g; Saturated Fat: 7.9g; Protein: 42.7g; Carbs: 6.9g; Fiber: 0.4g; Sugar: 0.8g*

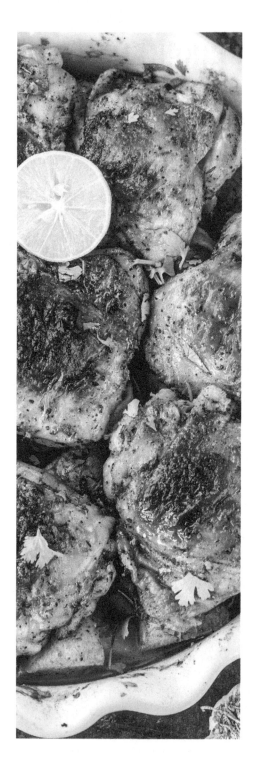

DIJON CHICKEN THIGHS

Preparation Time: 10 minutes
Cooking time: 50 minutes
Servings: 4

Ingredients:

- 1 ½ Lb. chicken thighs, skinless and boneless
- 4 Tbsp. maple syrup
- 2 Tsp. Olive oil
- 2 Tbsp. Dijon mustard
- ¼ cup French mustard

Directions:

1. Preheat the oven to 375 F/ 190 C.
2. In a mixing bowl, mix together maple syrup, olive oil, Dijon mustard, and French mustard.
3. Add chicken to the bowl & mix until chicken is well coated with maple mixture.
4. Arrange chicken in a baking dish and bake in preheated oven for 45-50 minutes.
5. Serve and enjoy.

Nutrition: *Calories: 401; Total Fat: 15.3g; Saturated Fat: 3.8g; Protein: 49.6g; Carbs: 13.8g; Fiber: 0.3g; Sugar: 12g*

DELICIOUS TACO CHICKEN

Preparation Time: 10 minutes
Cooking time: 6 hours
Servings: 4

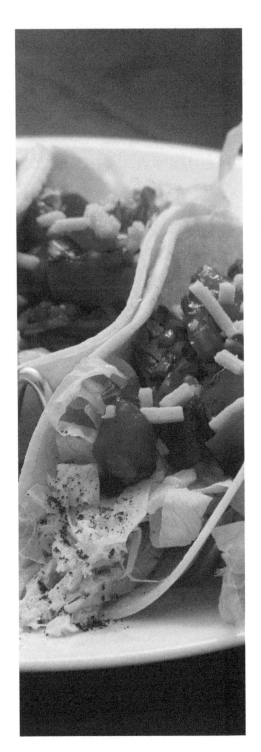

Ingredients:
- 1 Lb. chicken breasts, skinless and boneless
- 1 cup chicken broth
- 2 Tbsp. taco seasoning

Directions:
1. Place chicken in the slow cooker.
2. Mix together chicken broth and taco seasoning and pour over chicken.
3. Cover slow cooker w/ lid and cook on low for 6 hours.
4. Shred the chicken using a fork.
5. Serve and enjoy.

Nutrition: *Calories: 233; Total Fat: 8.7g; Saturated Fat: 2.4g; Protein: 34g;Carbs: 1.7g; Fiber: 0g; Sugar: 0.5g*

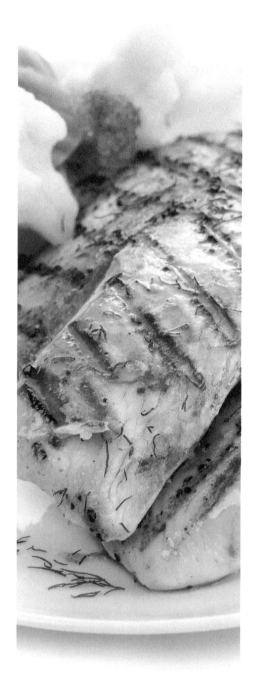

EASY BROILED FISH FILLET

Preparation Time: 10 minutes
Cooking time: 10 minutes
Servings: 2

Ingredients:

- 2 cod fish fillets
- 2 Tsp. Butter
- ¼ Tsp. Paprika
- 1/8 Tsp. Curry powder
- ½ Tsp. Sugar
- 1/8 Tsp. Pepper
- 1/8 Tsp. Salt

Directions:

1. Preheat the broiler.
2. Spray broiler pan w/ cooking spray and set aside.
3. In a small bowl, mix together paprika, curry powder, sugar, pepper, and salt.
4. Coat fish fillet with paprika mixture and place on broiler pan.
5. Broil fish in a preheated broiler for 10-12 minutes or until fish just begins to flakey.
6. Top with butter and serve.

Nutrition: *Calories: 129; Total Fat: 4.9g; Saturated Fat: 2.4g; Protein: 20.1g; Carbs: 1.3g; Fiber: 0.2g; Sugar: 1g*

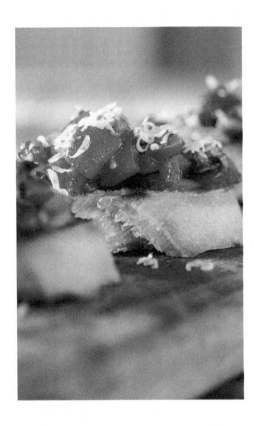

BAKED TOMATO BASIL FISH

Preparation Time: 10 minutes
Cooking time: 19 minutes
Servings: 2

Ingredients:
- 2 cod fillets
- 2 Tsp. Parmesan cheese, grated
- 2 tomatoes, sliced
- ¼ Tsp. Dried basil
- 1 Tsp. Olive oil
- 1 Tbsp. fresh lemon juice
- 1/8 Tsp. Pepper
- 1/8 Tsp. Salt

Directions:
1. Place fish fillets in greased baking dish.
2. Mix together oil and lemon juice and drizzle over fish fillets.
3. Season fish with basil, pepper, and salt.
4. Arrange tomato slices on top of fish fillets.
5. Sprinkle grated parmesan cheese on top.
6. Cover dish with foil and bake at 400 F/ 200 C for 10-12 minutes.
7. Serve and enjoy.

Nutrition: *Calories: 147; Total Fat: 4.4g; Saturated Fat: 0.9g; Protein: 22.2g; Carbs: 5g; Fiber: 1.5g; Sugar: 3.4g*

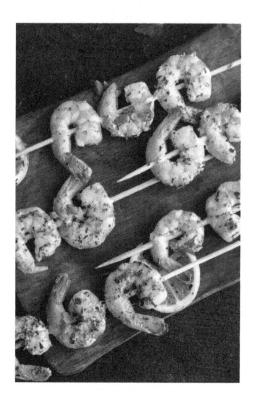

FLAVORFUL GRILLED SHRIMP

Preparation Time: 10 minutes
Cooking time: 6 minutes
Servings: 4

Ingredients:

- 1 Lb. shrimp, peeled and deveined
- 1 Tbsp. olive oil
- 1 ½ Tsp. Italian herb seasoning
- 1 ½ Tsp. Paprika
- 1 Tbsp. brown sugar
- ¼ Tsp. Pepper
- ½ Tsp. Salt

Directions:

1. In a small bowl, combine olive oil, brown sugar, paprika, Italian herb seasoning, pepper, and salt.
2. Add shrimp in a zip-lock bag and pour olive oil mixture over shrimp.
3. Seal bag & shake until shrimp is well coated—place in refrigerator overnight.
4. Thread shrimp onto soaked wooden skewers.
5. Preheat the grill to medium-high heat.
6. Place shrimp skewers on hot grill & cook for 2-3 minutes each side.
7. Serve and enjoy.

Nutrition: *Calories: 176; Total Fat: 5.5g; Saturated Fat: 1.1g; Protein: 26g;Carbs: 4.5g; Fiber: 0.3g; Sugar: 2.3g*

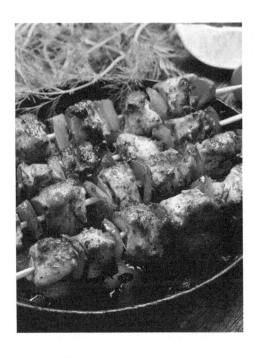

CHICKEN KABABS

Preparation Time: 10 minutes
Cooking time: 15 minutes
Servings: 4

Ingredients:
- 1 ½ Lb. chicken breasts, skinless, boneless, and cut into 1-inch cubes
- 1 Tbsp. olive oil
- 1 Tbsp. curry powder
- 1 Tbsp. brown sugar
- 2 Tbsp. peanut butter
- ½ cup soy sauce, low-sodium

Directions:
1. Add chicken in a large zip-lock bag.
2. Mix together soy sauce, olive oil, curry powder, brown sugar, and peanut butter and pour over chicken in a small bowl.
3. Seal bag then shakes until chicken is well coated.
4. Place in refrigerator overnight.
5. Thread marinated chicken onto soaked wooden skewers.
6. Preheat the grill on high.
7. Spray grill with cooking spray, then place chicken skewers on hot grill and cook for 12-15 minutes. Turn frequently.
8. Serve and enjoy.

Nutrition: *Calories: 431; Total Fat: 20.4g; Saturated Fat: 4.9g; Protein: 53.4g; Carbs: 7.1g; Fiber: 1.3g; Sugar: 3.5g*

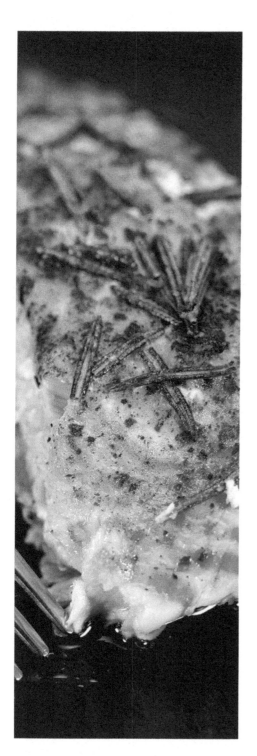

BAKED SALMON

Preparation Time: 10 minutes
Cooking time: 10 minutes
Servings: 6

Ingredients:
- 1 Lb. salmon
- 1 Tsp. Ginger, grated
- 2 ½ Tbsp. Dijon mustard
- 3 Tbsp. maple syrup
- 3 Tbsp. olive oil
- 1 Tsp. Pepper

Directions:
1. In a small bowl, mix olive oil, mustard, maple syrup, ginger, and pepper.
2. Preheat the oven to 400 F/ 200 C.
3. Spray a baking tray w/ cooking spray and set aside.
4. Place salmon on a baking tray and spread olive oil mixture over salmon evenly.
5. Bake in preheated oven for 10 minutes.
6. Serve and enjoy.

Nutrition: *Calories: 192; Total Fat: 12g; Saturated Fat: 1.7g;Protein: 15g;Carbs: 7.5g; Fiber: 0.3g; Sugar: 6g*

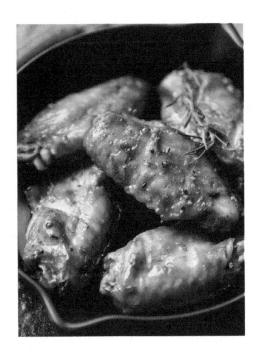

BAKED CHICKEN WINGS

Preparation Time: 10 minutes
Cooking time: 55minutes
Servings: 4

Ingredients:
- 2 Lbs. chicken wings
- 1 Tsp. Worcestershire sauce
- 2 Tbsp. butter
- 1/3 cup cayenne pepper sauce,
- ¼ cup flour, gluten-free
- Pepper
- Salt

Directions:
1. Preheat the oven to 400 F/ 200 C.
2. Line baking tray w/ parchment paper and set aside.
3. Add flour to the zip-lock bag. Season chicken w/ pepper and salt and add in a zip-lock bag.
4. Seal zip-lock bag and shake until chicken is coated with flour.
5. Place coated chicken wings on a baking tray and bake in preheated oven for 45-50 minutes. Turn halfway through.
6. Meanwhile, in a small saucepan, mix together Worcestershire sauce, butter, and cayenne pepper sauce. Bring to boil. Remove saucepan from heat & let it cool completely.
7. Place baked chicken wings in a large mixing bowl. Pour prepared sauce over chicken wings and toss well.
8. Serve and enjoy.

Nutrition: *Calories: 534; Total Fat: 23.9g; Saturated Fat: 8.5g; Protein: 67.3g; Carbs: 10.3g; Fiber: 2.2g; Sugar: 1g*

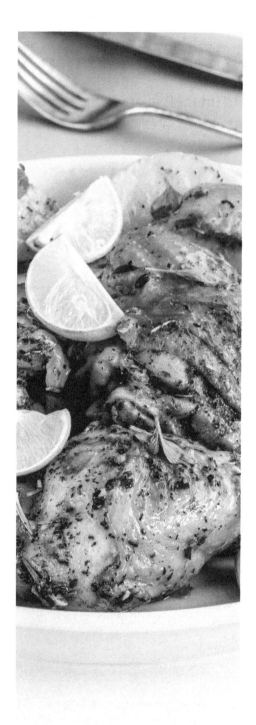

SPICY LEMON CHICKEN

Preparation Time: 10 minutes
Cooking time: 15 minutes
Servings: 6

Ingredients:

- 8 chicken thighs, skinless and boneless
- 1 Tbsp. fresh ginger, minced
- 1 ½ Tbsp. cayenne pepper
- 3 Tbsp. paprika
- ¼ cup olive oil
- 1 cup fresh lemon juice
- 1 Tsp. Salt

Directions:

1. In a large bowl, whisk the lemon juice, ginger, cayenne, paprika, olive oil, and salt.
2. Add chicken to the bowl and stir until well coated.
3. Place in refrigerator overnight.
4. Preheat the grill on high.
5. Place marinated chicken on hot grill & cook until done. Turn halfway through.
6. Serve and enjoy.

Nutrition: *Calories: 469; Total Fat: 23.9g; Saturated Fat: 5.6g; Protein: 57.4g; Carbs: 4.2g; Fiber: 1.9g; Sugar: 1.4g*

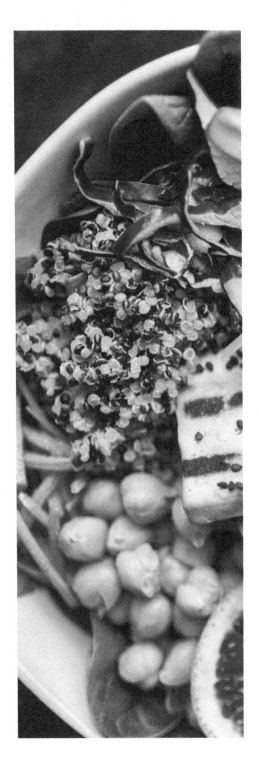

BOWL WITH CASHEW TAHINI SAUCE

Preparation Time: 10 minutes
Cooking time: 0 minutes
Servings: 2

Ingredients:

- 3/4 cup unsalted cashews
- 1/2 cup water
- 1/4 cup packed parsley leaves
- 1 tablespoon lemon juice or cider vinegar
- 1 tablespoon extra-virgin olive oil
- 1/2 teaspoon reduced-sodium tamari or soy sauce
- 1/4 teaspoon salt
- 1/2 cup cooked lentils
- 1/2 cup cooked quinoa
- 1/2 cup shredded red cabbage
- 1/4 cup grated raw beet
- 1/4 cup chopped bell pepper
- 1/4 cup grated carrot
- 1/4 cup sliced cucumber
- Toasted chopped cashews for garnishing (optional)

Directions:

1. In a blender, mix the tamari or soy sauce, cashews, salt, water, oil, lemon juice or vinegar, and parsley until a creamy consistency is reached.
2. Place the quinoa and lentils in the centre of a serving bowl; then, layer the remaining ingredients on top, clockwise from the outside of the bowl. Place 2 tablespoons of the cashew sauce on top of the vegetables, and set the remaining sauce aside for later use. You can sprinkle cashews on top if you'd like to.

Nutrition: *Calories: 361; Fat: 10g; Carbs: 54g; Fiber: 14g; Protein: 17g*

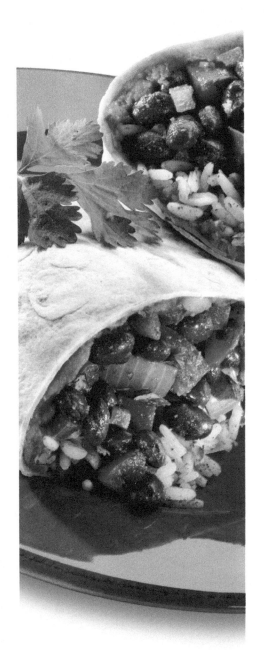

RICE BEAN FREEZER BURRITOS

Preparation Time: 10 minutes
Cooking time: 0 minutes
Servings: 8

Ingredients:

- 2 (15 ounces) cans low-sodium black or pinto beans, rinsed
- 4 teaspoons chili powder
- 1 teaspoon ground cumin
- 2 cups shredded sharp Cheddar cheese
- 1 cup chopped grape tomatoes
- 4 scallions, chopped
- 1/4 cup chopped pickled jalapeños
- 2 tablespoons chopped fresh cilantro
- 8 (8 inches) whole-wheat tortillas, at room temperature
- 2 cups cooked brown rice

Directions:

1. To make a nearly smooth mixture, mash the beans, cumin, and chilli powder combined in a big dish till the combination is almost completely smooth.
2. Stir in cilantro, jalapeños, scallions, tomatoes and cheese, then mix to blend.
3. Place approximately a ½ cup's worth of the filling on the lowest of each tortilla. Next, evenly spread approximately a quarter cup's worth of rice over the filling.
4. It should be rolled up tightly, and the ends should be tucked in as you proceed. Wrap each tortilla in a piece of aluminium foil. You have the option of freezing it for approximately three months.

Nutrition: *Calories: 401; Fat: 13g; Carbs: 53g; Fiber: 8g; Protein: 17g*

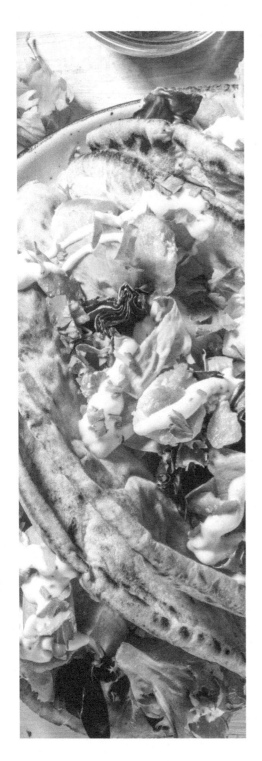

ROASTED VEGGIE HUMMUS PITA POCKETS

Preparation Time: 10 minutes
Cooking time: 0 minutes
Servings: 1

Ingredients:

- 1 (6 ½ inches) whole-wheat pita bread
- 4 tablespoons hummus
- 1/2 cup mixed salad greens
- 1/2 cup Sheet-Pan Roasted Root Vegetables, roughly chopped (see associated recipe)
- 1 tablespoon crumbled Feta cheese

Directions:

1. Halve the pita bread. Set the inside of each half of the pita pocket with 2 tablespoons of hummus.
2. Stuff with Feta, roasted vegetables, and greens on each pita pocket.

Nutrition: *Calories: 357; Fat:12g; Carbs: 54g; Fiber: 10g; Protein:14g*

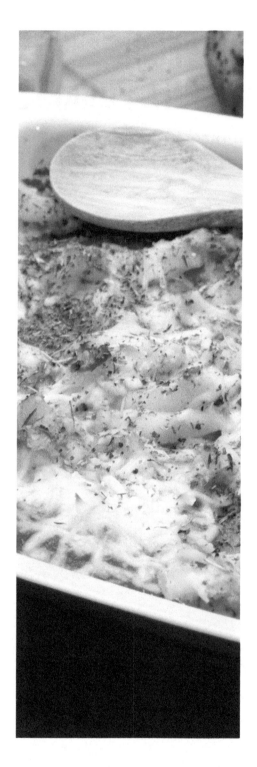

SAUSAGE PEPPERS BAKED ZITI

Preparation Time: 10 minutes
Cooking time: 30 minutes
Servings: 4

Ingredients:

- 8 ounces whole-wheat penne or ziti pasta
- 1 (16 ounces) bag frozen pepper and onion mix
- 6 ounces turkey sausage crumbled
- 2 (8 ounces) cans no-salt-added tomato sauce
- 1 teaspoon garlic powder
- 1 teaspoon dried oregano
- 1/4 teaspoon salt
- 1/2 cup reduced-fat Cottage cheese
- 3/4 cup Italian blend shredded cheese

Directions:
1. Make the pasta in accordance with the instructions provided on the compendium by placing it in a saucepan of water that is simmering. Strain.
2. In the meantime, put a big ovenproof skillet on the stove over medium-high heat.
3. After adding the sausage and frozen vegetables, linger cooking for an additional ten-fifteen mins, stirring the mixture regularly, until the majority of the liquid that was in the vegetables has evaporated.
4. Prepare the broiler while also positioning a tray in the uppermost portion of the oven.
5. Combine salt, oregano, garlic powder, and tomato sauce into the skillet.
6. Set the heat to medium-low; mix in the pasta and Cottage cheese.
7. Cook while stirring for around 2 minutes, till heated through.
8. Place shredded cheese on top.
9. Put the skillet on the broiler that has been warmed, and brown the cheese for one to two minutes.

Nutrition: *Calories: 408; Fat: 10g; Carbs: 8g; Fiber: 11g; Protein: 27g*

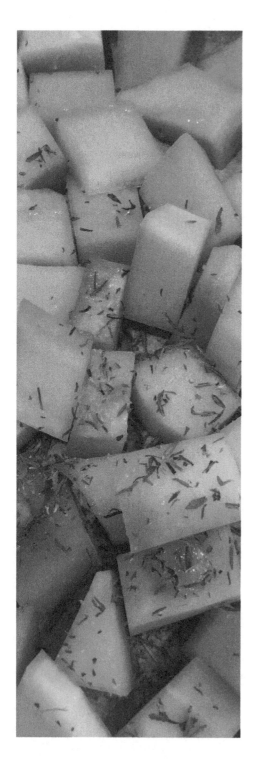

SAUTEED BUTTERNUT SQUASH

Preparation Time: 10 minutes
Cooking time: 15 minutes
Servings: 7

Ingredients:

- 1 large butternut squash (2-3 pounds), peeled, seeded and cubed
- 1 tablespoon extra-virgin olive oil

Directions:

1. Oil should be heated over a medium flame in a large pot.
2. Squash can be cooked for 15 minutes at a time with frequent turning until it starts to brown and softens.

Nutrition: *Calories: 75; Fat: 2g; Carbs: 15g; Fiber: 3g; Protein: 1g*

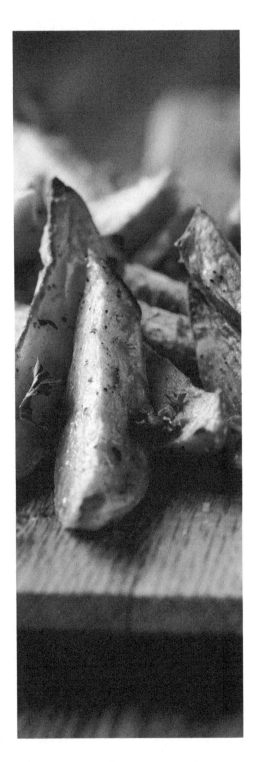

SPICED SWEET POTATO WEDGES

Preparation Time: 10 minutes
Cooking time: 20-30 minutes
Servings: 4

Ingredients:

- 2 (20 ounces) sweet potatoes, scrubbed
- 1 tablespoon olive oil
- 1 teaspoon packed brown sugar
- 1/4 teaspoon kosher salt
- 1/4 teaspoon smoked paprika
- 1/4 teaspoon black pepper
- 1/4 teaspoon pumpkin pie spice
- 1/4 teaspoon hot chili powder

Directions:

1. Prepare to preheat the oven to 425 degrees Fahrenheit.
2. Put a baking sheet into the oven so that it may get preheated.
3. Cut each sweet potato in half length, then cut each half into 8 wedges for a total of 16 wedges.
4. Sweet potato wedges should be placed in a large basin and then coated thoroughly with olive oil using a tossing motion.
5. In a small bowl, combine the chilli powder, pumpkin pie spice, black pepper, smoked paprika, kosher salt, and brown sugar. Stir to combine.
6. Sprinkle the spice mixture over the sweet potatoes, then toss to evenly coat the potatoes.
7. Place the wedges in a single layer on the baking tray that has been preheated.
8. Roast until it turns brown and soft, or for 25-30 minutes, flipping the wedges once halfway through the roasting time.

Nutrition: *Calories: 124; Fat: 3g; Carbs: 22g; Fiber: 3g; Protein: 2g*

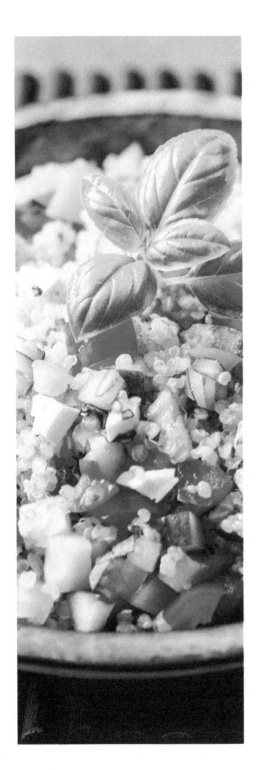

STETSON CHOPPED SALAD

Preparation Time: 10 minutes
Cooking time: 10 minutes
Servings: 1

Ingredients:

- 3/4 cup water
- 1/2 cup Israeli couscous
- 6 cups baby arugula
- 1 cup fresh corn kernels
- 1 cup halved or quartered cherry tomatoes
- 1 firm-ripe avocado, diced
- 1/4 cup toasted pepitas
- 1/4 cup dried currants
- 1/2 cup chopped fresh basil
- 1/4 cup buttermilk
- 1/4 cup mayonnaise
- 1 tablespoon lemon juice
- 1 small clove garlic, peeled
- 1/4 teaspoon salt
- 1/4 teaspoon ground pepper

Directions:

1. Bring a tiny amount of water to a boil in a saucepan.
2. After adding the couscous, decrease the temperature to maintain a slow boil, conceal, and continue cooking for 8-10 mins, or till all of the water is engrossed.
3. Transfer to a sieve with a fine-mesh screen, rinse under running cold water, and drain thoroughly.
4. On a serving plate, spread the arugula.
5. Put the arugula over the currants, pepitas, avocado, tomatoes, corn, and couscous in decorative lines.
6. Blend in a little food processor till all of the ingredients for the sauce (pepper, salt, garlic, lemon juice, mayonnaise, buttermilk, and basil) are completely smooth.
7. Just before you are ready to serve the salad, sprinkle it with the dressing.

Nutrition: *Calories: 376; Fat: 23g; Carbs: 39g; Fiber: 7g; Protein: 9g*

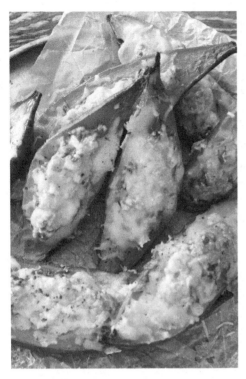

STUFFED SWEET POTATO WITH HUMMUS DRESSING

Preparation Time: 10 minutes
Cooking time: 15 minutes
Servings: 1

Ingredients:
- 1 large, sweet potato, scrubbed
- 3/4 cup chopped kale
- 1 cup canned black beans, rinsed
- 1/4 cup hummus
- 2 tablespoons water

Directions:
1. After making holes in the sweet potato all over again with a fork, insert it in the microwave and cook it on high for seven to ten minutes, or until it is fully cooked.
2. Rinse and drain the kale and let the water hold to the leaves. On medium-high heat, cook the kale in a medium saucepan, covered, until it wilts; stir 1-2 times.
3. Put in beans; pour 1-2 tablespoons of water if the pot dries.
4. Cook and stir occasionally without cover for 1-2 minutes until the mixture is steaming.
5. Break and open the sweet potato; add the beans and the kale mixture on top.
6. Combine two tbsp. of water with the hummus in a separate minor bowl. In order to achieve the desired consistency, add additional water if necessary.
7. Spread the hummus dressing on top of the sweet potato.

Nutrition: *Calories: 472; Fat: 1g; Carbs: 85g; Fiber: 22g; Protein: 21g*

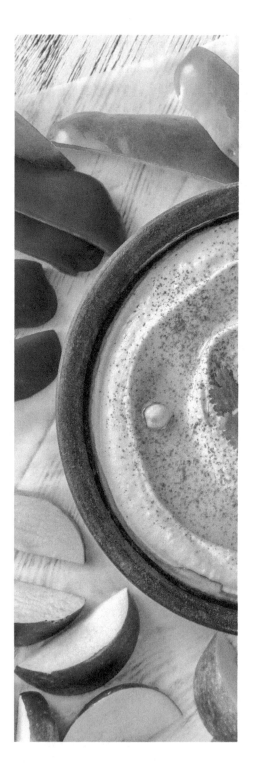

SWEET SAVORY HUMMUS PLATE

Preparation Time: 10 minutes
Cooking time: 0 minutes
Servings: 4

Ingredients:

- 3/4 cup white bean dip
- 1 cup green beans, stem ends trimmed
- 8 mini bell peppers
- 20 Castelvetrano olives
- 8 small watermelon wedges or 2 cups cubed watermelon
- 1 cup red grapes
- 20 gluten-free crackers
- 1/2 cup salted roasted pepitas
- 8 coconut-date balls

Directions:

1. Separate the items equally into 4 plates.
2. Serve with hard cider if desired.

Nutrition: *Calories: 654; Fat: 30g; Carbs: 84mg; Fiber: 11g; Protein: 14g*

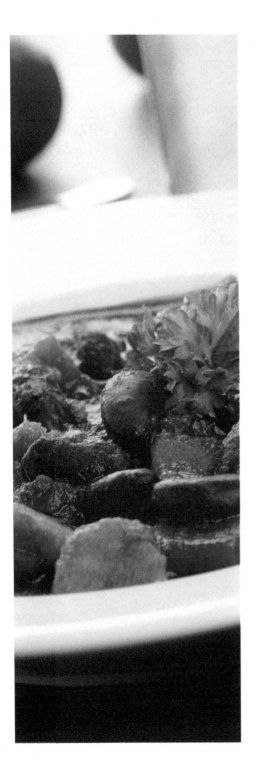

SWEET POTATO BLACK BEAN CHILI FOR TWO

Preparation Time: 10 minutes
Cooking time: 20 minutes
Servings: 2

Ingredients:

- 2 teaspoons virgin olive oil
- 1 small onion
- 1 small, sweet potato
- 2 garlic cloves
- 1 tablespoon chili powder
- 2 teaspoons ground cumin
- 1/4 teaspoon ground chipotle Chile
- 1/8 teaspoon salt, or to taste
- 1 1/3 cup water
- 1 (15 ounces) can black beans, rinsed
- 1 cup canned diced tomatoes
- 2 teaspoons lime juice
- 2 tablespoons chopped fresh cilantro

Directions:

1. After heating a large skillet with oil at medium temperature, include the potato and onion, and continue to cook while turning often for approximately four minutes, until either the onion gets somewhat softer.
2. After adding the salt, chipotle, cumin, chilli powder, and garlic, continue stirring while cooking for approximately 30 seconds until the mixture becomes aromatic.
3. After attaching the water, fetch it up to a simmer, at that point conceal it and decrease the temperature so that it continues to gently simmer.
4. Cook until the potato becomes tender, around 10-12 minutes.
5. Toss in the tomato paste and beans after adding the lime juice and put the mixture to a boil, stirring often.
6. After four minutes, decrease the temperature to preserve a boil and continue cooking the mixture until it has greatly reduced in size.

Nutrition: *Calories: 365; Fat: 7g; Carbs: 67g; Fiber: 18g; Protein: 14g*

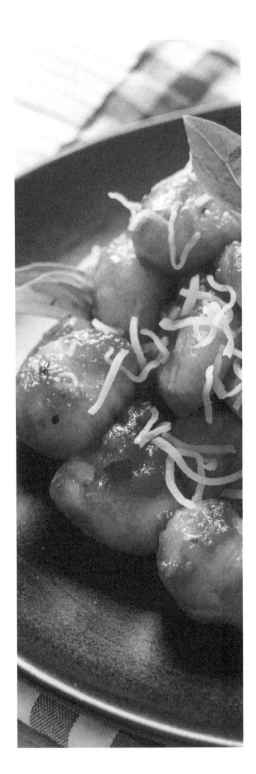

TOMATO ARTICHOKE GNOCCHI

Preparation Time: 10 minutes
Cooking time: 20 minutes
Servings: 4

Ingredients:

- 2 tablespoons extra-virgin olive oil
- 1 (16 ounces) package shelf-stable gnocchi
- 1 small onion, sliced
- 1 small red bell pepper
- 4 large garlic cloves
- 1 tablespoon chopped fresh oregano
- 1 (15 ounces) can chickpeas
- 1 (14 ounces) can no-salt-added diced tomatoes
- 1 (9 ounces) box frozen artichoke hearts
- 8 pitted Kalamata olives, sliced
- 1 tablespoon red-wine vinegar
- 1/4 teaspoon ground pepper

Directions:

1. One tablespoon of oil should be heated over medium-high heat in a skillet that does not stick.
2. Place the gnocchi in the saucepan and bake them, mixing them frequently, for about five mins, or until they have puffed up and begun to brown.
3. Put them in a dish and cover it to keep them at a warm temperature.
4. Try the temperature down to moderate. Include the chopped onion as well as the residual tbsp of oil in the dish.
5. Cook for two to three minutes, swirling the pan occasionally, until the mixture starts to turn golden.
6. After adding the bell pepper, continue cooking for about three minutes, swirling the pan occasionally, until the pepper is crisp-tender.
7. After incorporating the oregano and garlic, continue to stir-fry the mixture for another half a minute.
8. Include the artichokes, tomatoes, and chickpeas; cook for approximately three mins while mixing irregularly, or till the vegetables are warm.
9. Mix in the gnocchi, pepper, vinegar, and olives.
10. Sprinkle oregano on top, if desired.

Nutrition: *Calories: 427; Fat: 11g; Carbs: 71g; Fiber: 10g; Protein: 12g*

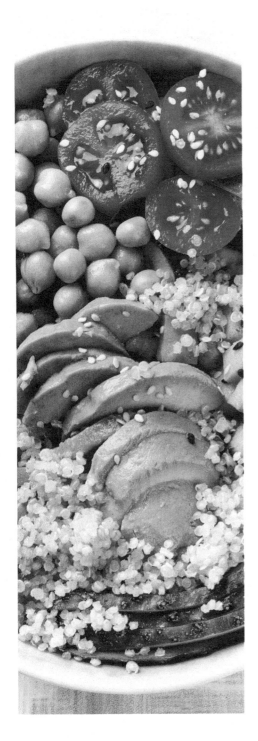

VEGAN BUDDHA BOWL

Preparation Time: 10 minutes
Cooking time: 20 minutes
Servings: 4

Ingredients:
- 1 medium sweet potato
- 3 tablespoons extra-virgin olive oil
- 1/2 teaspoon salt
- 1/2 teaspoon ground pepper
- 2 tablespoons tahini
- 2 tablespoons water
- 1 tablespoon lemon juice
- 1 small clove garlic
- 2 cups cooked quinoa
- 1 (15 ounces) can chickpeas, rinsed
- 1 firm-ripe avocado, diced
- 1/4 cup cilantro or parsley

Directions:

1. To begin preheating the oven, adjust the temperature to 425 degrees Fahrenheit.
2. In a larger bowl, combine the sweet potato mash with 1/4 teaspoon salt, 1/4 teaspoon pepper, and 1 tablespoon oil.
3. Add a rim to a baking sheet. Toss the vegetables in the oven and bake for fifteen–eighteen mins, mixing once, until they are tender.
4. Mix together the other 2 tbsp olive oil, the lemon juice, the tahini, the garlic, and the remaining 1/4 teaspoon salt and 1/4 teaspoon of pepper in a small container. Mix thoroughly.
5. Split the quinoa among 4 bowls to serve.
6. To finish, sprinkle on a garnish of chickpeas, sweet potato, and avocado in equal parts.
7. Tahini sauce should be drizzled over the top.
8. Finish with some chopped parsley or cilantro.

Nutrition: *Calories: 455; Fat: 25g; Carbs: 51g; Fiber: 11g; Protein: 11g*

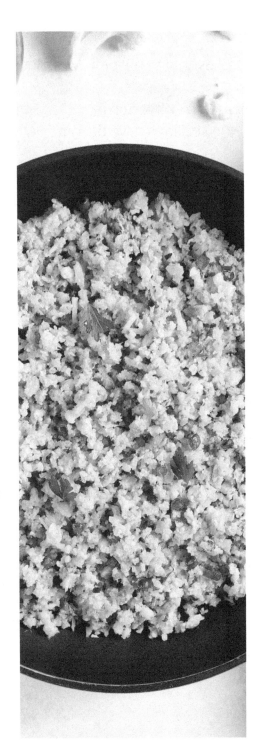

VEGAN CAULIFLOWER FRIED RICE

Preparation Time: 10 minutes
Cooking time: 15 minutes
Servings: 4

Ingredients:

- 3 tablespoons peanut oil, divided
- 3 scallions, sliced
- 1 tablespoon grated fresh ginger
- 1 tablespoon minced garlic
- 1/2 cup diced red bell pepper
- 1 cup trimmed and halved snow peas
- 1 cup shredded carrots
- 1 cup frozen shelled edamame, thawed
- 4 cups riced cauliflower
- 1/3 cup unsalted roasted cashews
- 3 tablespoons tamari or soy sauce
- 1 teaspoon toasted sesame oil

Directions:

1. One tablespoon of peanut oil should be heated over high heat in a wok or a standard cooking pan.
2. Cook the ginger, garlic, and scallions in the heated oil while stirring constantly for thirty to forty seconds, or until the scallions have become more tender.
3. Add the snow peas, bell pepper, edamame, and carrots then cook while stirring for 2-4 minutes until just tender.
4. Move everything to a dish or plate.
5. Place in the pan the two remaining teaspoons of peanut oil.
6. Cauliflower should be cooked in oil for about two minutes, stirring it occasionally, until it is mostly softened.
7. Place the vegetables back in the skillet, and then stir in the cashews, tamari or soy sauce, and sesame oil.
8. Mix thoroughly until everything is thoroughly combined.

Nutrition: *Calories: 287; Fat: 19g; Carbs: 18g; Fiber: 6g; Protein: 10g*

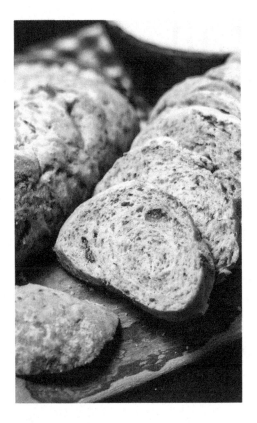

OATMEAL BREAD TO LIVE FOR

Preparation Time: 10 minutes
Cooking time: 30 minutes
Servings: 12

Ingredients:

- 1 ¼ cup (295 ml) water
- 2 teaspoons (10 ml) canola oil
- 1 tablespoon (15 g) brown sugar
- 1 cup (80 g) quick-cooking oats
- 2 ¼ cups whole-wheat flour, divided
- 1 tablespoon vital wheat gluten
- 1 ¼ teaspoon yeast
- 1 tablespoon shelled sunflower seeds

Directions:

1. Put water, oil, and sugar in the bread machine.
2. Add the oats and let them sit for 5 minutes.
3. Pour in two cups or 240 grammes of flour, as well as the gluten.
4. Make a hole in the centre of the flour where you may put the yeast.
5. Turn on the bread machine. (Use a setting for 1 ½-pound [680 g] loaf, dark if you have it). If the dough seems too sticky, add some flour as needed.
6. Add the sunflower seeds to the beep.

Nutrition: *Calories: 287; Fat: 19g; Fiber: 6g; Carbs: 18g; Protein: 8g*

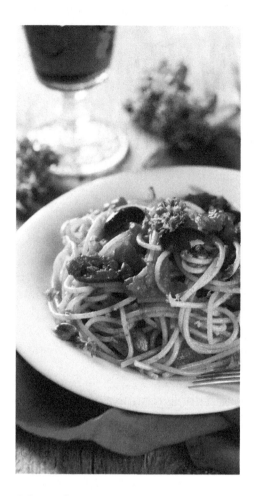

VERMICELLI PUTTANESCA

Preparation Time: 10 minutes
Cooking time: 15 minutes
Servings: 6

Ingredients:

- 4 large tomatoes
- 1/4 cup chopped flat-leaf parsley
- 16 large black olives
- 3 tablespoons capers
- 4 anchovy fillets
- 2 tablespoons olive oil
- 3 large garlic cloves
- 1/2 teaspoon ground pepper
- 1-pound whole-wheat vermicelli, or spaghettini
- 1/4 cup freshly grated Pecorino Romano

Directions:

1. Combine pepper, garlic, oil, anchovies, capers, olives, parsley, and tomatoes in a large pasta serving bowl.
2. While you're waiting for the sauce to simmer, start the pasta by boiling a big kettle of salted water. The pasta should be cooked for about eight to ten mins, depending on the packet.
3. After draining the pasta, place it in the bowl where the sauce is being kept.
4. Next, give everything a good shake to mix it up.
5. After that, taste it and adjust the seasoning as necessary.
6. Cheese should be dusted on top, and it should be served right away.

Nutrition: *Calories: 379; Fat: 10g; Carbs: 64g; Fiber: 11g; Protein: 14g*

SPINACH AND ARTICHOKE DIP PASTA

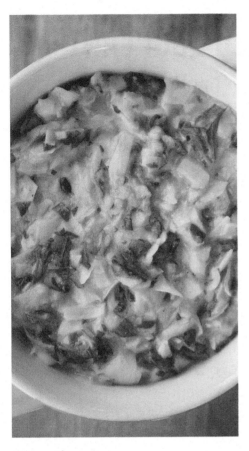

Preparation Time: 10 minutes
Cooking time: 15 minutes
Servings: 4

Ingredients:

- Whole-wheat rotini – 8 ounces
- Baby spinach – 5 ounces, chopped
- Cream cheese – 4 ounces, low-fat, cut into chunks
- Milk – ¾ cup, low-fat
- Parmesan cheese – ½ cup, grated
- Garlic powder – 2 tsp
- Ground pepper – ¼ tsp
- Artichoke hearts – 14 ounces, rinsed, squeezed dry and chopped

Directions:

1. Add water into the saucepan and boil it. Add pasta and cook it. Then, drain it.
2. Cook the spinach in the pot by combining it with the one tablespoon of water and cooking it over a medium flame. Cook for another minute, or until the greens have wilted.
3. Move it to the bowl we have prepared. In a saucepan, combine the milk and cream and give it a good whisking.
4. Pepper, garlic powder, and parmesan cheese should then be added, and the mixture should be cooked until it has thickened. After draining the spinach, add it to the sauce along with the artichoke and pasta. Cook it well.
5. Serve and enjoy!

Nutrition: *Calories: 371; Fat: 9.1g; Carbs: 56.1g; Fiber: 7.9g; Protein: 16.6g*

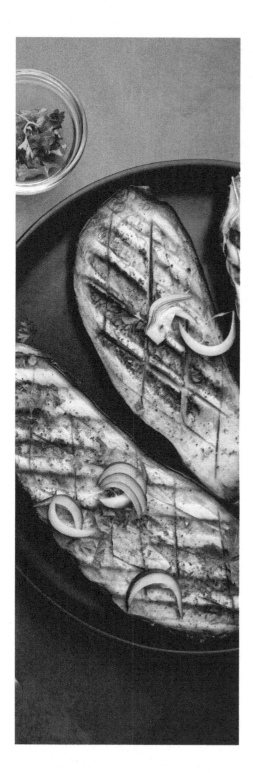

GRILLED EGGPLANT

Preparation Time: 5 minutes
Cooking time: 40 minutes
Servings: 4

Ingredients:

- Water – 4 cups
- Cornmeal – 1 cup
- Butter – 1 tbsp
- Salt – ½ tsp
- Plum tomatoes – 1 lb, chopped
- Extra-virgin olive oil – 4 tbsp
- Fresh oregano – 2 tsp, chopped
- Garlic – 1 clove, grated
- Ground pepper – ½ tsp
- Crushed red pepper – ¼ tsp
- Eggplant – 1 ½ lbs., cut into half-inch-thick slices
- Feta cheese – ¼ cup, crumbled
- Fresh basil – ½ cup, chopped

Directions:

1. Add water into the saucepan and boil it over high flame.
2. Mix it thoroughly after you add the cornmeal. After that, decrease the temperature and linger to cook for another 35 mins, or till the meat is soft.
3. When it is finished, take it away from the flame. After adding the salt and butter, make sure to mix everything well.
4. During this time, get the grill ready by preheating it over medium-high heat.
5. To the bowl, add tomatoes, salt, crushed red pepper, pepper, garlic, oregano, and three tablespoons of oil, then mix everything together thoroughly.
6. Eggplant should be rubbed with one tablespoon of oil, placed on the grille, and cooked for four mins on individual sideways. Please allow it to cool for ten minutes.
7. Add it to the tomatoes.
8. Sprinkle with fresh basil leaves.
9. Place vegetable mixture over the polenta and top with cheese.

Nutrition: *Calories: 354; Fat: 20.6g; Carbs: 39g; Fiber: 8.4g; Protein: 6.8g*

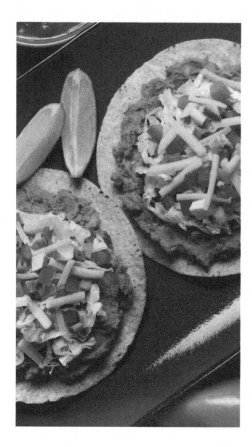

TEX-MEX BEAN TOSTADAS

Preparation Time: 10 minutes
Cooking time: 15 minutes
Servings: 4

Ingredients:

- Tostada shells – 4
- Pinto beans – 16 ounces, rinsed and drained
- Salsa – ½ cup, prepared
- Chipotle seasoning – ½ tsp
- Cheddar cheese – ½ cup, shredded
- Iceberg lettuce – 1 ½ cups
- Tomato – 1 cup, chopped
- Lime wedges – 1

Directions:

1. Turn the oven up to 350 degrees Fahrenheit.
2. Bake the tostada shells for three to five minutes after placing them on the baking pan.
3. Meanwhile, mix the seasoning; salsa, and bean into the bowl.
4. Use a potato masher to blend the ingredients together.
5. The bean mixture should next be distributed evenly among the tostada shells.
6. Place one piece of the cheese on top. Cook for five mins.
7. Top with chopped tomato and shredded lettuce.
8. Then, place the remaining cheese and lime wedges.

Nutrition: *Calories: 230, Fat: 6g; Carbs: 33g; Fiber: 6g; Protein: 12g*

CHAPTER SIX:
Desserts

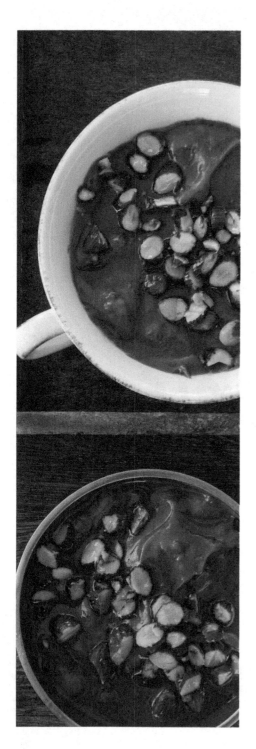

MILLET CHOCOLATE PUDDING

Preparation Time: 10 minutes
Cooking time: 0 minutes
Servings: 4

Ingredients:
- 1 Lb. cooked millet
- 2 cup unsweetened almond milk
- ½ medium banana
- ¼ cup of cocoa powder
- 2 tablespoons maple syrup

Directions:
1. Pour all ingredients in a blender and then pulse until smooth.
2. Pour the chocolate mixture into bowls and allow to set in the fridge before serving.

Nutrition: *Calories: 260, Total Fat 5.8g, Saturated Fat 2.9g, Total Carbs 45.9g, Net Carbs 42.4g, Protein 8.9g, Sugar: 14.3g, Fiber: 3.5g*

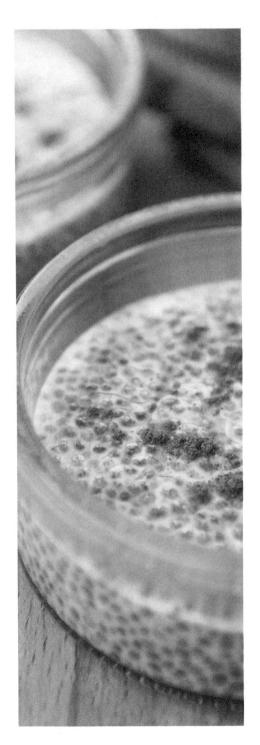

VANILLA MAPLE CHIA PUDDING

Preparation Time: 10 minutes
Cooking time: 0 minutes
Servings: 1

Ingredients:
- 3 tablespoons chia seeds
- 1 cup of coconut milk
- ½ teaspoon vanilla extract
- 1 tablespoon maple syrup

Directions:
1. Mix all ingredients in a container and stir until well combined.
2. Place inside the fridge and allow to set overnight.

Nutrition: *Calories: 280, Total Fat 12.6g, Saturated Fat 5.1g, Total Carbs 31.7g, Net Carbs 26.5g, Protein 10.2g, Sugar: 24.2g, Fiber: 5.2g*

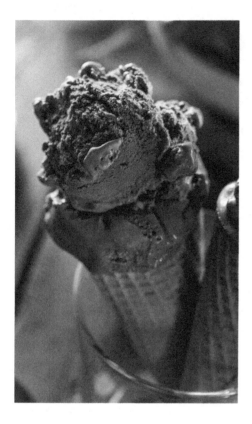

DARK CHOCOLATE GELATO

Preparation Time: 10 minutes
Cooking time: 10 minutes
Servings: 16

Ingredients:

- 2 ¼ cups of coconut milk
- ¾ cup lactose-free heavy cream
- 2 tablespoons arrowroot starch
- ½ cup of cocoa powder
- 4 Oz. dark chocolate
- What you'll need from the store cupboard:
- ¾ cup of sugar

Directions:

1. In a saucepan, place half of the coconut milk, cream, arrowroot starch, cocoa powder, and dark chocolate. Add in the sugar.
2. Turn on the stove & bring the mixture to a simmer until it thickens. Turn off the heat and add the remaining milk. Mix until well combined.
3. Pour into an ice cream maker. Turn the ice cream maker for 3 hours until the mixture turns into a gelato.
4. If you do not have an ice cream maker, you can place the mixture in a lidded container. Place in the fridge for 8 hrs. But make sure that you mix the mixture every hour to create the creamy gelato texture.

Nutrition: *Calories: 145, Total Fat 11.4g, Saturated Fat 9.1g, Total Carbs 11g, Net Carbs 7.5g, Protein 2.5g, Sugar: 3.4g, Fiber: 3.5g, Sodium: 20mg, Potassium: 299mg*

BREAD PUDDING WITH BLUEBERRIES

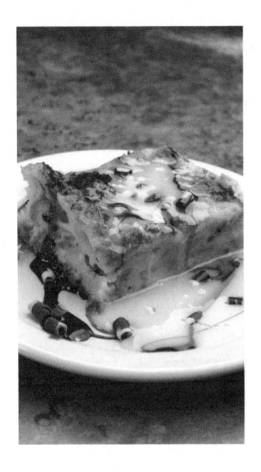

Preparation Time: 10 minutes
Cooking time: 40 minutes
Servings: 2

Ingredients:
- 1 extra-large egg
- 2/3 cup unsweetened almond milk
- 1 tablespoon maple syrup
- ¼ teaspoon vanilla extract
- 4 slices of gluten-free bread
- ½ cup blueberries
- A dash of ground cinnamon
- What you'll need from the store cupboard:
- None

Directions:
1. Preheat the oven to 3750F.
2. In a bowl, almond milk, whisk the eggs, and maple syrup until well combined. Add in the vanilla extract.
3. Cut the crusts from the bread & slice the bread into tiny cubes. Place the bread cubes in a greased baking dish and pour the egg mixture. Top with blueberries and sprinkle with a dash of cinnamon.
4. Bake for 40 minutes or until the egg mixture is set and the top has browned and puffed up.

Nutrition: *Calories: 268, Total Fat 6.5g, Saturated Fat 2.6g, Total Carbs 44.9g, Net Carbs 42.8g, Protein 7.8g, Sugar: 25.6g, Fiber: 2.1g, Sodium: 238mg, Potassium: 215mg*

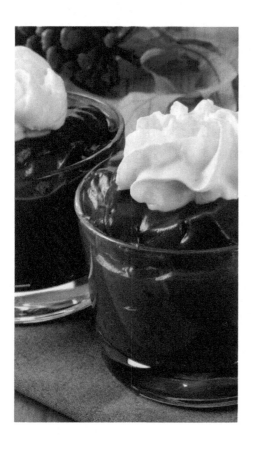

CHOCOLATE ENGLISH CUSTARD RECIPES

Preparation Time: 10 minutes
Cooking time: 10 minutes
Servings: 2

Ingredients:

- 1 ½ tablespoon tapioca starch
- 1 egg
- 1 tablespoon pure maple syrup
- ¾ cup almond milk
- 1 tablespoon water
- 1 ½ tablespoon cocoa powder
- What you'll need from the store cupboard:
- None

Directions:

1. Add all ingredients in a saucepan and whisk until all lumps are removed.
2. Place the saucepan on the stove and then bring to a boil over low heat while stirring constantly.
3. Turn off the heat once the mixture thickens.
4. Pour into ramekins and refrigerate for 3 hours before serving.

Nutrition: *Calories: 170, Total Fat 6.5g, Saturated Fat 2.1g, Total Carbs 24.6g, Net Carbs 21.4g, Protein 5.8g, Sugar: 16.2g, Fiber: 3.2g, Sodium: 340mg, Potassium: 892mg*

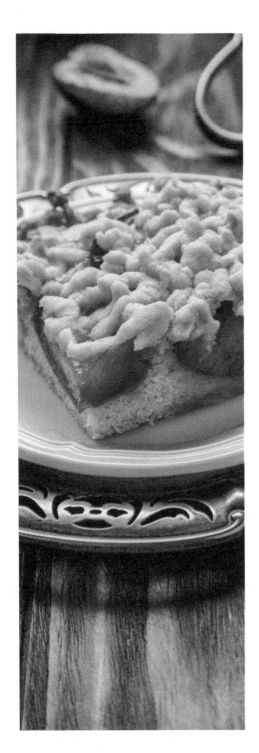

BERRY CRUMB CAKE

Preparation Time: 20 minutes
Cooking time: 50 minutes
Servings: 16

Ingredients:
- 2 cups gluten-free flour
- 1 teaspoon baking powder
- ¾ cup butter, cold
- ¾ cup of coconut milk
- 1 tablespoon lemon juice
- 2 eggs
- 1 cup strawberries and blueberries
- What you'll need from the store cupboard:
- 1 cup of sugar

Directions:

1. Preheat the oven to 3500F and lightly grease an 8x8 square pan.
2. In a bowl, add the sugar, baking powder, and sugar.
3. Add butter into the flour mixture gradually. Use a pastry blender until you achieve a crumb-like texture—Reserve half of the crumb mixture for the topping.
4. In another bowl, stir in the coconut milk, and lemon juice. Let it stand for 5 minutes.
5. Add into half of the flour mixture the eggs and milk and mix until well combined.
6. Fold in the berries.
7. Pour the mixture into the prepared pan & sprinkle on top of the reserved crumb topping.
8. Bake for 50 minutes.
9. Allow cooling before slicing.

Nutrition: *Calories: 171, Total Fat 12.7g, Saturated Fat 8.2g, Total Carbs 13.6g, Net Carbs 13g, Protein 1.9g, Sugar: 10.1g, Fiber: 0.6g, Sodium: 107mg, Potassium: 70mg*

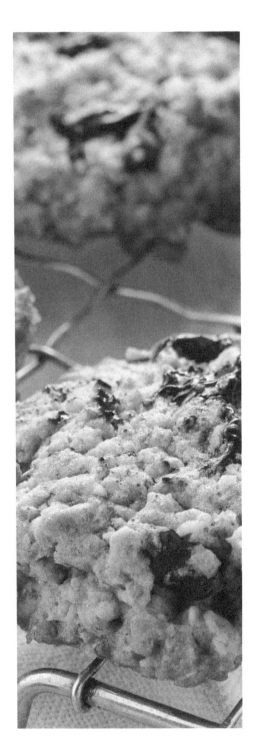

PEANUT BUTTER OATMEAL CHOCOLATE CHIP COOKIES

Preparation Time: 20 minutes
Cooking time: 15 minutes
Servings: 14

Ingredients:

- 1 cup gluten-free flour
- ½ teaspoon xanthan gum
- 1 teaspoon baking soda
- 8 tablespoons unsalted butter, cold and cubed
- ½ cup natural creamy peanut butter
- 2/3 cup sugar
- 1 teaspoon pure vanilla extract
- 1 large egg
- ¾ cup gluten-free quick oats
- 1 cup semi-sweet mini chocolate chips
- What you'll need from the store cupboard:
- ¼ teaspoon salt

Directions:

1. Preheat the oven to 3500F. Line a baking sheet with parchment paper.
2. Mix together the gluten-free flour, xanthan gum, baking soda, and salt in a bowl.
3. In another bowl, cream the butter and add in the peanut butter, sugar, and vanilla extract. Beat in the eggs & continue to beat until well-combined.
4. Gradually add the dry ingredients and mix until everything is incorporated.
5. Stir in the oats, chocolate chip cookies. Scoop the cookie dough & place it on the cookie sheet.
6. Bake for 12 minutes.
7. Remove from the cookie sheet on the cooling rack before serving.

Nutrition: *Calories: 199, Total Fat 10.3g,Saturated Fat 3.9g, Total Carbs 25.5g, Net Carbs 23.6, Protein 4.2g, Sugar: 15.8g, Fiber: 1.9g, Sodium: 65mg, Potassium: 161mg*

GRANOLA BARS

Preparation Time: 15 minutes
Cooking time: 15 minutes
Servings: 12

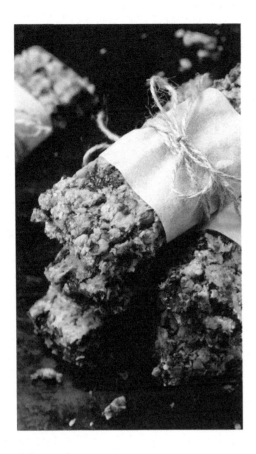

Ingredients:
- 1 cup rice flake
- 1 cup millet flakes
- ½ cup dried cranberries
- ½ cup pumpkin seeds
- ¼ cup sunflower seeds
- ½ cup peanut butter
- 2 teaspoons malt syrup
- 1 teaspoon cinnamon powder
- What you'll need from the store cupboard:
- Coconut oil for greasing

Directions:
1. Preheat the oven to 3550F and grease a small baking tray.
2. In a bowl, mix together the rice flakes, millet, cranberries, pumpkin seeds, and peanut butter.
3. In a blender, mix together the peanut butter, and malt syrup. Add in the cinnamon powder.
4. Pour into the granola mixture & mix well.
5. Press into the baking tray and bake for 15 minutes.
6. Allow hardening before cutting into bars.

Nutrition: *Calories: 180, Total Fat 8.6g, Saturated Fat 1.4g, Total Carbs 23.4g, Net Carbs 19g, Protein 6.1g, Sugar: 4.4g, Fiber: 4.4g, Sodium: 175mg, Potassium: 270mg*

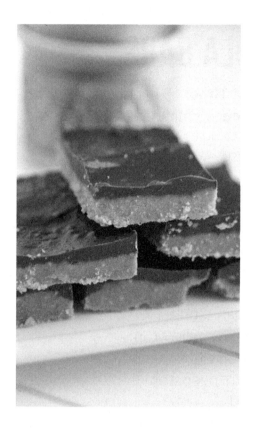

BAKED PEANUT BUTTER PROTEIN BARS

Preparation Time: 20 minutes
Cooking time: 0 minutes
Servings: 12

Ingredients:

- 1 cup natural creamy peanut butter
- ¾ cup maple syrup
- 1 teaspoon vanilla bean paste
- 1 ½ cups gluten-free rolled oats
- 1 cup of protein powder
- What you'll need from the store cupboard:
- None

Directions:

1. Line a baking pan with parchment paper.
2. In a microwave-safe bowl, heat the peanut butter and maple syrup for 30 seconds. Stir then add in the vanilla bean paste then heat again for 30 seconds.
3. Stir in oats and protein powder.
4. Spread into the prepared pan and press using the back of the spoon.
5. Refrigerate for an hour and cut into 12 bars.

Nutrition: *Calories: 271, Total Fat 14.9g, Saturated Fat 2.5g, Total Carbs 27.6g, Net Carbs 23.4g, Protein 14g, Sugar: 13.7g, Fiber: 4.2g, Sodium: 128mg, Potassium: 442mg*

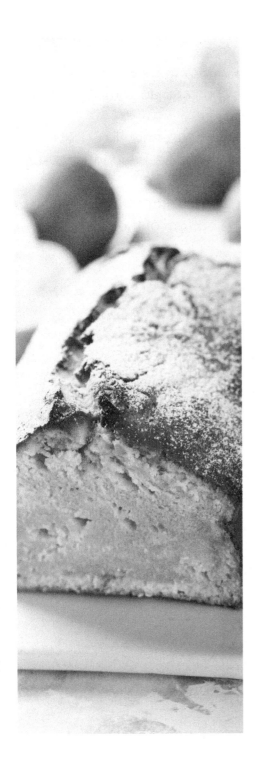

LIME CAKE

Preparation Time: 20 minutes
Cooking time: 45 minutes
Servings: 8

Ingredients:

- 2 ½ cups gluten-free flour
- 1 tablespoon baking powder
- 1 teaspoon xanthan gum
- 4 large eggs
- 1 cup canola oil
- 1 cup of coconut milk
- 1 teaspoon vanilla extract
- 1 teaspoon lime extract
- What you'll need from the store cupboard:
- 2 cups of sugar
- ½ teaspoon salt
- 1 tablespoon lime zest
- 3 tablespoons freshly squeezed lime juice

Directions:

1. Preheat the oven to 3500F and grease a cake pan with shortening or oil.
2. In a large bowl, baking powder, mix the flour, and xanthan gum. Sift through a sieve to aerate the dry ingredients.
3. In another bowl, mix together the eggs, canola oil, coconut milk, vanilla extract, lime extract, sugar, salt, lime zest, and lime juice. Beat until the sugar dissolves, and the liquid turns smooth.
4. Fold in the dry ingredients gradually and mix until the lumps are removed.
5. Pour the batter into the prepared pan. Tap the bottom of the pan to remove too much air within the batter.
6. Place in the oven and bake for 45 minutes.

Nutrition: *Calories: 422, Total Fat 30.7g, Saturated Fat 3.4g, Total Carbs 35.2g, Net Carbs 34.9g, Protein 3.1g, Sugar: 26.5g, Fiber: 0.3g, Sodium: 221mg, Potassium: 114mg*

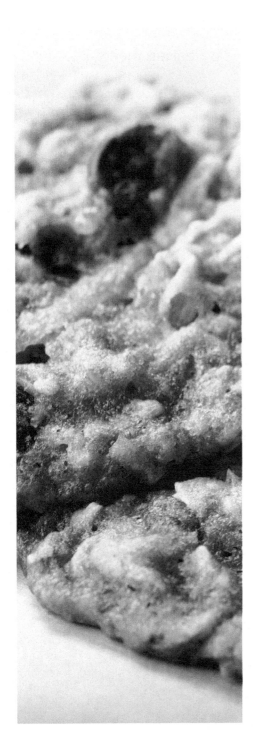

BANANA OATMEAL CHOCOLATE CHIP COOKIES (HEALTHY!)

Preparation Time: 15 minutes
Cooking time: 12 minutes
Total time: 27 minutes
Servings: 18

Ingredients:

- Two cups quick oats
- ½ cups almond flour
- 3 large brown bananas mashed (about 1 cup)
- ½ cup light brown sugar or palm sugar
- Large egg
- Two teaspoons of baking powder
- One teaspoon vanilla extract
- ¼ teaspoon salt
- ¼ cups dark chocolate chips

Directions:

1. Preheat the oven to 350 degrees fahrenheit. 2 big baking sheets, lined with parchment paper
2. Combine the oats, almond flour, mashed bananas, brown sugar, egg, baking powder, vanilla extract, and salt in an electric stand mixer bowl. Beat the mixture until it is smooth and uniform.
3. Then, with the mixer on low, fold in half of the chocolate chips.
4. To distribute the cookies onto the baking pans, use a 1.5 tablespoon cookie scoop. Set them apart by 2 inches.
5. Place 4-5 chocolate chips on top of each cookie, flattening the dough balls slightly.
6. Bake for 12 minutes or until the edges are firm. Cool for 5 minutes on the cookie sheets before transferring.

Nutrition: *Calories: 4192, Carbohydrates: 24 g, Protein: 51 g, Fat: 9 g, Cholesterol: 261 mg*

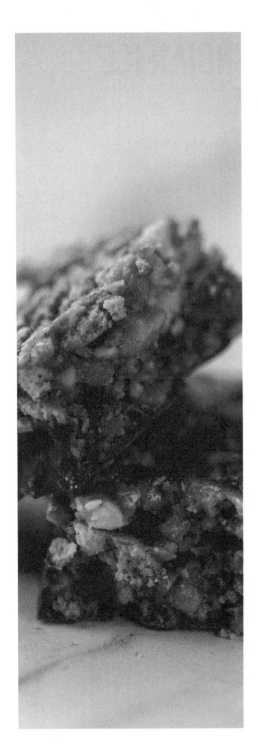

LARABAR SNACK BAR

Preparation Time: 5 minutes
Cooking time: 5 minutes
Total time: 10 minutes
Servings: 12

Ingredients:

- 2 cup raw almonds
- 3/4 cup pitted dates packed
- 1 cup dried unsweetened apples
- 1/4 cup raisins packed
- 1/2 teaspoon cinnamon
- 1/4 teaspoon sea salt

Directions:

1. In a food processor, combine all of the ingredients and process until finely chopped and sticky.
2. Line an 8-inch baking dish with wax paper, leaving enough to hang over the sides to cover the mixture. Fill the dish halfway with the mixture and top with wax paper. Press or roll out the ingredients until it is smooth.
3. Remove the wax paper and bars from the pan and cut them into 12 equal bars. Wrap each piece in wax paper and store it in an airtight container.

Nutrition: *Calories: 153, Carbohydrates: 17 g, Protein: 17 g, Fat: 27 g, Cholesterol: 89 mg*

KULFI INDIAN ICE CREAM

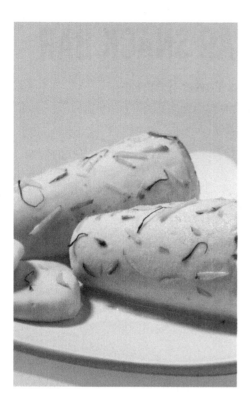

Preparation Time: 10 minutes
Cooking time: 160 minutes
Total time: 170 minutes
Servings: 16

Ingredients:

- 2 cups heavy cream
- 14 ounces can sweeten condensed milk
- 2 teaspoon ground cardamom
- 1 teaspoon vanilla extract
- ½ cup chopped pistachios
- 1 pinch saffron + 1 tbs warm water

Directions:

1. In a small dish, combine 1 tablespoon hot tap water. Allow a pinch of saffron to soak to absorb its color and taste.
2. Meanwhile, prepare an electric mixer fitted with a whip attachment. Pour in the heavy cream, cardamom powder, and vanilla essence. Whip the mixture at high speed until firm peaks form.
3. Using a rubber spatula, scrape the bowl. Then add the saffron and water and mix well.
4. Fold in the sweetened condensed milk using a spatula. Fold in the chopped pistachios after the mixture is smooth and uniform.
5. Insert the kulfi in an airtight container and freeze it, or spoon it into tiny cups for popsicles and place a popsicle stick in the center of each one.
6. Freeze for a minimum of 3 hours.

Nutrition: *Calories: 200, Carbohydrates: 16g, Protein: 14 g, Fat: 18 g, Cholesterol: 44 mg*

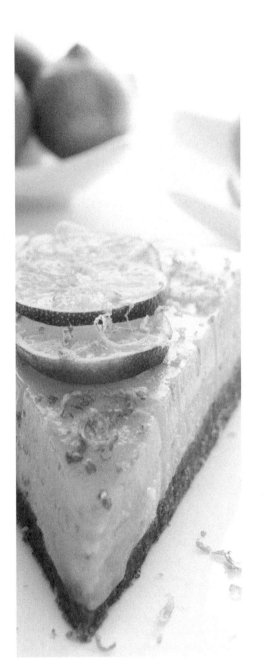

EASY NO-BAKE KEY LIME PIE RECIPE

Preparation Time: 20 minutes
Cooking time: 240 minutes
Total time: 260
Servings: 8

Ingredients:

For the graham cracker crust
- 12 whole graham crackers crushed (about 1 ½ cups)
- Six tablespoons melted butter
- ¼ cup granulated sugar
- ¼ teaspoon salt

For the key lime pie filling
- Eight ounce cream cheese softened
- 14 ounce sweetened condensed milk
- ½ cup key lime juice
- 3-5 drops lime green food coloring if desired
- 8 ounce cool whip
- Lime zest for garnish

Directions:

1. Prepare a 9-inch pie pan as well as a food processor. In a food processor, combine the graham crackers. Close the lid and pulse into a fine crumb. After that, stir in the melted butter, sugar, and salt. To mix, pulse the ingredients together.

2. Fill the pie pan halfway with the graham cracker crumble. Press it into an equal layer over the bottom and up the edges of the pan with your hands. Keep refrigerated until ready to use.

3. Wipe the food processor bowl clean. Then combine the cream cheese, sweetened condensed milk, and lime juice in a mixing bowl. Blend until smooth. (if wanted, add food coloring here.)

4. Take the food processor blade out of the machine. Scoop the cool whip into the lime mixture and stir well. Fold the cool whip into the mixture with a spatula until completely smooth.

5. Fill the pie crust with the filling. Then, store the mixture in the freezer for at least 4 hours, undisturbed.

6. If preferred, top with fresh lime zest when ready to serve. While still frozen, cut into pieces. Allow each piece to remain at room temperature for 10 minutes before serving somewhat softened.

Nutrition: *Calories: 451, Carbohydrates: 60 g, Protein: 63 g, Fat: 28 g, Cholesterol: 59 mg*

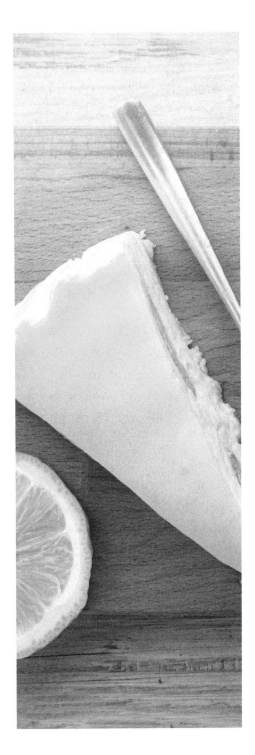

LEMON CHEESECAKE RECIPE (LIMONCELLO CAKE!)

Preparation Time: 20 minutes
Cooking time: 60 minutes
Total time: 80 minutes
Servings: 16

Ingredients:

For the biscoff crust
- 8.8 oz biscoff cookies, 1 package
- 1/2 cup granulated sugar
- 1/2 teaspoon salt
- 1/2 cup unsalted butter, melted

For the limoncello cheesecake filling
- 24 oz cream cheese, softened
- 4 large eggs
- 3/4 cup granulated sugar
- 1 large lemon, zested and juiced (1/4 cup juice)
- 1/4 cup limoncello liqueur
- 1/2 teaspoon vanilla extract
- 1/2 teaspoon salt

For the sour cream topping
- 16 oz sour cream
- 1/4 cup granulated sugar
- 3 tablespoons limoncello liqueur

Directions:

1. Preheat the oven to 350 degrees fahrenheit. Place one oven rack in the center and one at the bottom of the oven. To catch any spillage, use a big rimmed baking sheet on the bottom rack. Preheat the oven to 350°f. Line the bottom of a 9 1/2-inch springform pan with parchment paper. Then, securely tighten the ring around the bottom. (if desired, trim the paper edges.)

2. To make the crust: in a food processor, combine the biscoff cookies, sugar, and salt. Pulse the cookies until they are finely ground. After that, add the melted butter and pulse to the mix. Fill the prepared pan halfway with the crust mixture. With your hands, press the crumbs all over the bottom of the pan and approximately two-thirds of the way up the edges. 10 minutes in the oven

3. Meanwhile, prepare the limoncello cheesecake filling by placing the cream cheese in the bowl of an electric mixer. 2 minutes on high to soften and fluff the cream cheese. Add the eggs one at a time, delaying adding another until the preceding egg is thoroughly mixed in. Using a spatula, scrape the bowl. Then mix in the other ingredients until fully smooth—bake for 45 minutes after pouring the filling into the crust.

4. To make the sour cream topping, combine the sour cream, sugar, and limoncello in a medium mixing bowl and whisk until smooth. Once the cheesecake has baked and is nearly set in the center, pour the sour cream filling over the top and return to the oven for 10-12 minutes.

5. 1 hour on the counter to cool the cheesecake. Then place in the refrigerator for at least 3 hours to cool. Remove the ring from the springform pan and place the cheesecake on a cake plate. Cut into slices and serve chilled.

Nutrition: *Calories: 386, Carbohydrates: 35 g, Protein: 55 g, Fat: 17 g, Cholesterol: 108 mg*

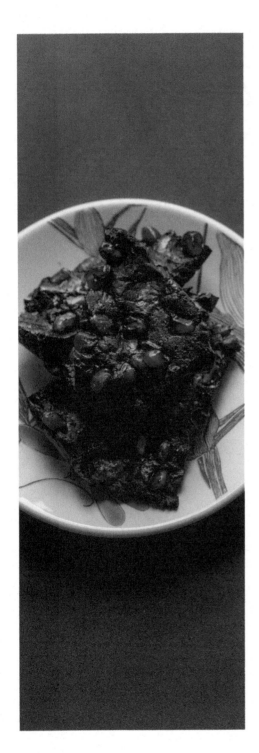

DARK CHOCOLATE WITH POMEGRANATE SEEDS

Preparation Time: 10 minutes
Cooking time: 2-3 minutes
Servings: 3

Ingredients:

- 150 g dark chocolate (at least 70% cocoa)
- 120 g pomegranate seeds (from 1 pomegranate)
- 1 teaspoon sea salt

Directions:

1. Scatter a layer of pomegranate seeds in a muffin tin (or muffin paper).
2. Melt the chocolate in the microwave.
3. Pour the chocolate into a bag, then cut a tiny hole so that it can be spread over the seeds. Add a layer of seeds and another of chocolate.
4. Sprinkle with a pinch of salt and chill in the refrigerator until the mixture is hard.
5. Enjoy cold.

Nutrition: *Calories: 82 Carbs: 19 g Protein: 1.9 g Fat: 0.2 g Sugar: 3.9 g Sodium: 37 mg Fiber: 3.7 g*

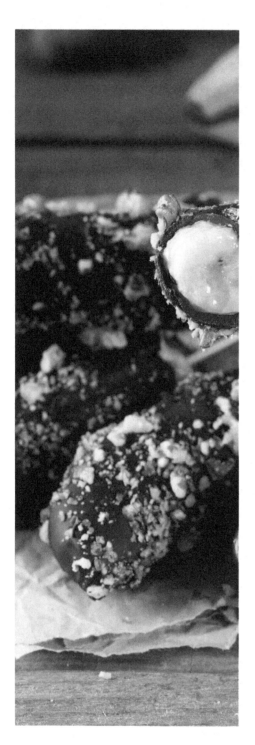

CHOCOLATE BUTTER HONEY COVERED BANANAS

Preparation Time: 10 minutes
Cooking time: 0 minutes
Servings: 3

Ingredients:

- 3 bananas
- 1 tablespoon oat bran
- 2 tablespoons cashew or almond butter
- 1 cup melted dark chocolate
- 1 tablespoon honey
- 1 teaspoon chia seeds
- 1 teaspoon cinnamon

Directions:

1. Mix the oat bran, seeds and cinnamon in a shallow bowl.
2. Mix the nut butter with honey.
3. Coat the bananas with nut butter and then add to the dry mixture so that they are coated on both sides.

Nutrition: *Calories: 11 Carbs: 3 g Protein: 0 g Fat: 0 g Sugar: 2.9 g Sodium: 0 mg Fiber: 0.1 g*

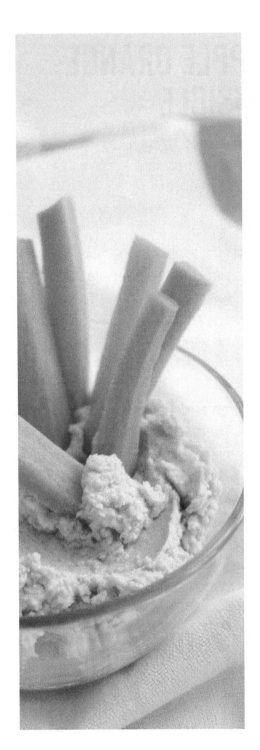

HUMMUS WITH TAHINI AND TURMERIC

Preparation Time: 10 minutes
Cooking time: 0 minutes
Servings: 4

Ingredients:
- 2 cans chickpeas, drained
- 50 ml lemon juice
- 60 ml tahini
- 1 garlic clove, minced
- 2 tablespoons extra-virgin olive oil
- 1/2 tablespoon turmeric powder
- 1/2 teaspoon sea salt

Directions:
1. Mix the tahini and lemon juice with olive oil, garlic, turmeric and salt for about 30 seconds using a hand blender or kitchen utensil.
2. Add the chickpeas and puree, making sure that no chickpeas remain unmixed on the sides. Pound until a uniform mixture is obtained.
3. Garnish with paprika powder and enjoy with any snacks, such as vegetable sticks.

Nutrition: *Calories: 33 Carbs: 8.1 g Protein: 0.2 g Fat: 0.1 g Sugar: 7.6 g Sodium: 130 mg Fiber: 0.1 g*

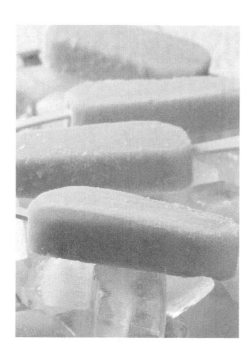

PINEAPPLE ORANGE CREAMSICLE

Preparation Time: 10 minutes
Cooking time: 12 minutes
Total time: 22 minutes
Servings: 10

Ingredients:
- Two cups of orange-pineapple juice
- One cup heavy cream
- ½ cup granulated sugar
- 2 teaspoons vanilla extract

Directions:
1. In a microwave-safe bowl, combine 1/2 cup juice and 1/2 sugar. Warm the juice for 1-2 minutes or until the sugar melts. Then add the remaining juice and whisk to combine.
2. Pour the heavy cream, vanilla extract, and 1 1/4 cup of the sweetened juice into a separate dish (or measuring pitcher). Stir everything together thoroughly. Then divide the mixture evenly among ten regular popsicle molds.
3. For 1 hour, place the popsicles in the freezer. Then, drizzle the remaining juice over the tops of each popsicle and insert wooden popsicle sticks. Freeze for at least 3 hours more.

Nutrition: *Calories: 145, Carbohydrates: 15 g, Protein: 17 g, Fat: 8 g, Cholesterol: 76 mg*

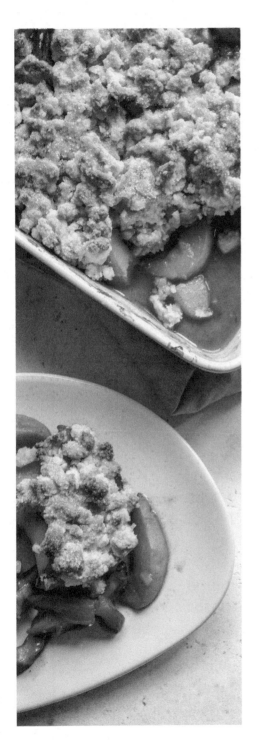

EASY PEACH COBBLER RECIPE WITH BISQUICK

Preparation Time: 10 minutes
Cooking time: 60 minutes
Total time: 70 minutes
Servings: 7

Ingredients:

- 48 oz fresh or frozen sliced peaches 6 ½ cups, with or without peels
- Two cups granulated sugar
- ½ teaspoon of pumpkin pie spice or apple pie spice blend
- Cups bisquick baking mix
- 1 cup of whole milk
- 1 cup of melted butter

Directions:

1. Preheat the oven to 350 degrees fahrenheit. Prepare a 9-by-13-inch baking dish and a large mixing basin.
2. If you are using fresh peaches, cut them into wedges and remove the pits. Fill the baking dish halfway with fresh (or frozen) peach slices. Then, over the peaches, add 1 cup sugar and the pumpkin pie spice. Toss the peach to coat it, then spread it out in an equal layer.
3. Combine the remaining 1 cup sugar, bisquick, and milk in a mixing basin. Whisk everything together well. Then add the melted butter and stir until combined.
4. Pour the batter over the peaches in an equal layer. Bake for 55- 60 minutes, depending on the size of the baking dish.
5. After 40 minutes, check on the cobbler. If the top begins to darken, loosely cover with foil and continue baking.
6. Allow at least 15 minutes for the cobbler to cool before serving. Serve in dishes with vanilla ice cream or whipped cream.

Notes: you don't like peaches? Replace the nectarines, plums, pitted cherries, or berries with an equal number of nectarines, plums, pitted cherries, or berries in this recipe.

How to keep leftovers: once the cobbler has completely cooled, cover it in plastic wrap or move it to a container with a lid. The fruit cobbler may be stored in the refrigerator for up to 4-5 days.

To put on ice: cook according to the recipe in a freezer-safe baking dish, cool, and cover the entire dish in plastic wrap. Wrap in tin foil and place in the freezer for up to 3 months. Unwrap and bake in a 350°f oven for 40-50 minutes, or until boiling.

Nutrition: *Calories: 420, Carbohydrates: 59 g, Protein: 11 g, Fat: 20 g, Cholesterol: 172 mg*

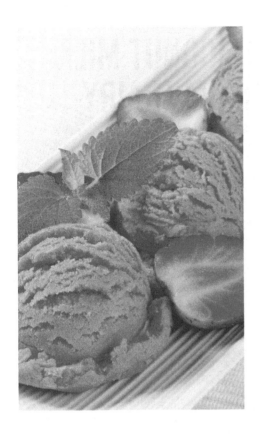

HEALTHY 5-MINUTE STRAWBERRY PINEAPPLE SHERBET

Preparation Time: 5 minutes
Cooking time: 5 minutes
Total time: 10 minutes
Servings: 16

Ingredients:

- One pound frozen strawberries
- One pound has frozen pineapple chunks
- 1/2 cups plain greek yogurt
- 1/2 cup honey or palm syrup
- Two teaspoon vanilla extract
- Pinch salt

Directions:

1. In a large food mixer, combine all of the ingredients. Pulse the frozen fruit to break it up. Then purée until completely smooth.
2. Serve immediately as soft serve, or freeze in an airtight container. Thaw for 15 minutes before scooping and serving if frozen.

Notes: This sherbet has a distinct honey taste. If you dislike the flavor of honey, use palm syrup.

Nutrition: *Calories: 70, Carbohydrates: 16 g, Protein: 2 g, Fat: 1 g, Cholesterol: 1 mg*

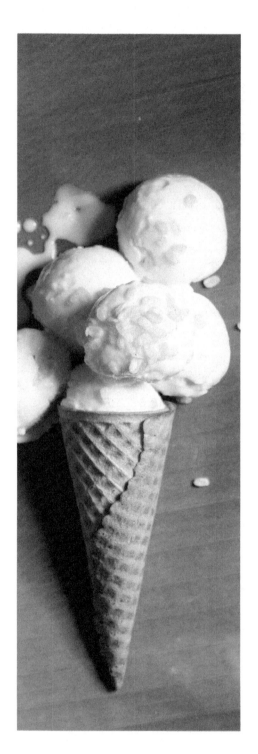

BEST COCONUT MILK ICE CREAM (DAIRY-FREE!)

Preparation Time: 3 minutes
Cooking time: 30 minutes
Total time: 33 minutes
Servings: 16

Ingredients:

- 27 ounce canned full-fat unsweetened coconut milk 2 cans
- 13.6 ounce can coconut cream
- One cup granulated sugar
- Two teaspoons of vanilla extract or vanilla bean paste
- ¼ teaspoon salt

Directions:

1. After making this ice cream numerous times, i learned that it does not always need to be heated/cooked before churning... This saves a huge amount of time. (this depends on the kind of coconut milk/cream and the kind of blender you use.) Put all ingredients in a blender and purée until smooth to see whether your ice cream has to be cooked. If the coconut ice cream mixture is smooth and free of clumps, you may churn it without heating.

2. Heat and stir: if there are any pieces of coconut cream in the recipe, they will freeze as hard waxy clumps in the ice cream. In this scenario, cook the mixture over medium heat until smooth, stirring often. Before churning, chill and cool to at least room temperature. * if you don't want to test the no-heat approach, simply combine all ingredients in a saucepot and cook over medium heat until smooth, allowing the coconut clumps and sugar to dissolve. Then take a break.

3. Set out a 1.5-2 quart ice cream machine after the ice cream mixture has cooled. Turn on the machine and place the frozen bowl inside. Fill the machine halfway with the extremely smooth ice cream mixture. Cook for 20-25 minutes, or until the mixture is thick, hard, and smooth.

4. Serve right away, or transfer to an airtight container and freeze until ready to use.

Nutrition: *Calories: 224, Carbohydrates: 16 g, Protein: 2 g, Fat: 19 g, Cholesterol: 27 mg*

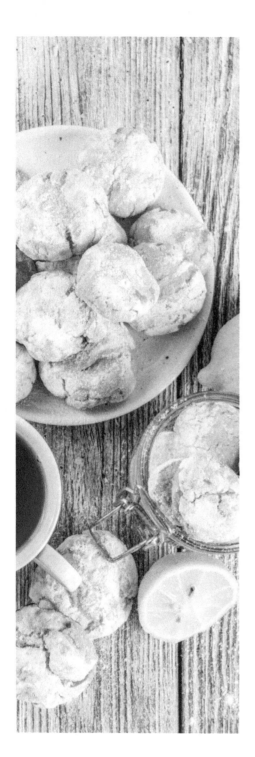

LEMON CRINKLE COOKIES RECIPE

Preparation Time: 15 minutes
Cooking time: 10 minutes
Total time: 25 minutes
Servings: 45

Ingredients:

- 1 cup unsalted butter, softened (2 sticks)
- ¾ cups granulated sugar
- 4 large eggs
- 2 tablespoons fresh lemon juice
- 2 tablespoon lemon zest
- 1 teaspoon vanilla extract
- 1 cup all-purpose flour (stir, spoon into the cup, and level)
- 2 teaspoon baking powder
- 1/2 teaspoon salt
- 1/4 teaspoon baking soda
- 2-5 drops yellow food coloring (optional)
- 2 cup powdered sugar

Directions:

1. In the bowl of an electric stand mixer, combine the butter and granulated sugar. Cream the butter and sugar together on high for 3-5 minutes, or until light and creamy. Using a rubber spatula, scrape the bowl.
2. Mix in the eggs, lemon juice, lemon zest, and vanilla extract at low speed. Scrape the bowl once more. Mix in 1 cup of flour, baking powder, salt, baking soda, and food coloring on low. Once mixed, gently fold in the remaining 2 cups of flour until smooth. (be careful not to overwork the dough!)
3. Refrigerate the dough for at least 30 minutes, covered. (the longer the dough is chilled, the puffier the cookies.) Preheat the oven to 375 degrees Fahrenheit. Set aside several baking sheets lined with parchment paper.
4. Set out a small dish of powdered sugar once the dough has cooled. To separate the dough into balls, use a 1 tablespoon cookie scoop. Roll each ball in powdered sugar, then place 2 inches apart on baking pans. (be careful to cover the cookies with powdered sugar generously.) You should not shrug them off.)
5. 9-10 minutes, or until the sides are golden brown and the middle appears slightly under baked. Allow them to cool on the baking pans so that the centers continue to bake as they cool.

Note: Storage suggestions: store the cookies in an airtight jar at room temperature. Consume within 7-10 days.

Citrus substitutions: In place of the lemon, you can use lime or orange juice and zest. You may also combine lemon and lime for a unique taste combination!

Nutrition: *Calories: 111, Carbohydrates: 16 g, Protein: 29 g, Fat: 18 g, Cholesterol: 63 mg*

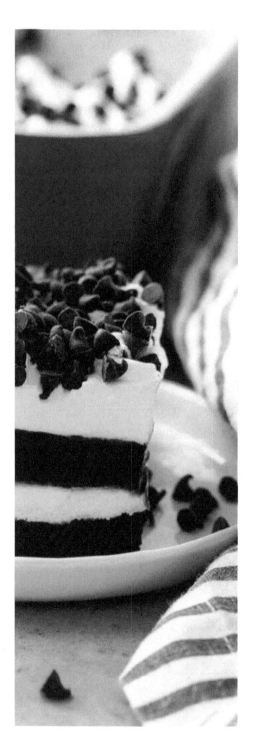

THE BEST NO-BAKE CHOCOLATE LASAGNA

Preparation Time: 20 minutes
Cooking time: 120 minutes
Total time: 140 minutes
Servings: 12

Ingredients:
Oreo layer
- 40 oreo cookies
- 7 tablespoons melted butter
- Cream cheese layer –
- 8 oz cream cheese softened
- 3 tablespoons granulated sugar
- Two tablespoons of milk
- 16 oz of cool whip reserve half for later

Chocolate pudding layer
- 7.8 oz instant chocolate pudding mix two small boxes
- 2 ¾ cups of milk
- Two teaspoons instant coffee granules
- Whipped topping layer –
- Remaining cool whip
- 2 cup mini chocolate chips or ½ cup chocolate shavings

Directions:

1. Set up a big food processor to make the oreo crust. In a mixing dish, combine the oreo cookies. Cover and pulse until tiny crumbs form. Then, pulse in the melted butter to coat. * if you don't have a food processor, you may smash the cookies with a rolling pin in a zip bag. Then, for the remaining processes, use a mixer.
2. Fill a 9 x 13 inch baking dish halfway with oreo crumbs. Chill after pressing into a uniform layer.
3. A layer of cream cheese: next, rinse off the food processor bowl. Combine the cream cheese, sugar, and milk in a mixing bowl. Blend until smooth. Then, using a knife, spoon half (8 oz) of the cool whip into the cream cheese. Fold the mixture with a spatula until it is smooth. Spread the mixture evenly over the crust in the baking dish. Chill.
4. Rinse the food processor bowl once more for the chocolate pudding layer. Combine the chocolate pudding powder, milk, and instant coffee in a mixing bowl. Puree till smooth, covered. In the baking dish, evenly distribute the ingredients.
5. Toppings: top the chocolate pudding with the remaining 8 oz of cool whip. Then, over the top, sprinkle with tiny chocolate chips or chocolate shavings.
6. Place in the refrigerator for at least 4 hours, covered. Freeze for 2-3 hours for optimum cutting results, then cut and serve. Allow 10-15 minutes for the frozen plated pieces to come to room temperature before serving.

Note: This is a fantastic make-ahead dessert that can be made 4-5 days ahead of time and stored in the freezer for up to 3 months.

Nutrition: *Calories: 533, Carbohydrates: 72 g, Protein: 16 g, Fat: 8 g, Cholesterol: 42 mg*

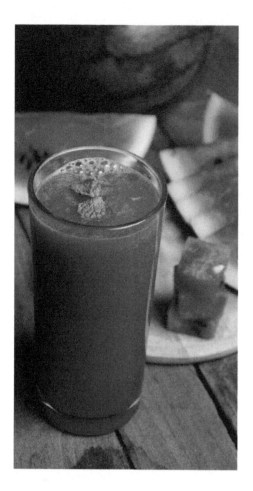

EASIEST HEALTHY WATERMELON SMOOTHIE RECIPE

Preparation Time: 3 minutes
Cooking time: 3 minutes
Total time: 6 minutes
Servings: 4

Ingredients:

- 4 cups fresh ripe watermelon cubes from a less melon
- 2 cup strawberry yogurt regular or a dairy-free variety
- 4 cups ice
- 1-2 tablespoons granulated sugar optional (only needed if the watermelon isn't very sweet.)

Directions:

1. In a blender, combine the watermelon cubes and yogurt. Puree till smooth, covered. Taste to see if more sugar is required.
2. Pour in the ice cubes (and sugar if desired). After that, cover and purée until smooth.
3. Serve right away.

Note: Garnish with cubes or slices of watermelon or cut strawberries.

Nutrition: *Calories: 120, Carbohydrates: 27 g, Protein: 27 g, Fat: 19 g, Cholesterol: 47 mg*

CHAPTER SEVEN:

21-Day Meal Plan

21-DAY MEAL PLAN

Day 1:
Breakfast: Gut-Healing Smoothie ..*page 34*
Snacks: Tangy Tomato Soup ..*page 2*
Lunch: Mushroom & Beef Bone Broth ..*page 72*
Snacks: Good-For-You Chocolate Chip Cookies ..*page 10*
Dinner: Cheeseburger Macaroni ..*page 112*
Dessert: Millet Chocolate Pudding ..*page 154*

Day 2:
Breakfast: Aloe-Mint Smoothie ..*page 35*
Snacks: Oat And Wheat Cookies ..*page 3*
Lunch: Shiitake-Miso Cod Soup ..*page 74*
Snacks: Oatmeal Sunflower Bread ..*page 11*
Dinner: Salmon Skewers ..*page 114*
Dessert: Vanilla Maple Chia Pudding ..*page 155*

Day 3:
Breakfast: Cinnamon Berry Smoothie ..*page 36*
Snacks: Maple Oatmeal Bread ..*page 5*
Lunch: Vegetable-Coconut Curry Soup ..*page 76*
Snacks: Southwest Stuffed Avocado Bowls ..*page 12*
Dinner: Lemon Chicken ..*page 115*
Dessert: Dark Chocolate Gelato ..*page 156*

21-DAY MEAL PLAN

Day 4:
Breakfast: Spinach and Aloe Smoothie ..*page 37*
Snacks: German Dark Bread ..*page 6*
Lunch: Deviled Egg Salad ..*page 78*
Snacks: Flaxseed Yogurt ..*page 14*
Dinner: Dijon Chicken Thighs ..*page 116*
Dessert: Bread Pudding with Blueberries ..*page 157*

Day 5:
Breakfast: Berry Flax Smoothie ..*page 38*
Snacks: Onion And Garlic Wheat Bread ..*page 7*
Lunch: Carrot and Beet Coleslaw ..*page 79*
Snacks: Raw Lemon Pie Bars ..*page 15*
Dinner: Delicious Taco Chicken ..*page 117*
Dessert: Chocolate English Custard Recipes ..*page 158*

Day 6:
Breakfast: Strawberry Healthy Gut Smoothie ..*page 39*
Snacks: White Chocolate-Cranberry Cookies ..*page 8*
Lunch: Hearty Winter Salad with Forbidden Rice ..*page 80*
Snacks: Trail-Mix Energy Bars ..*page 16*
Dinner: Easy Broiled Fish Fillet ..*page 118*
Dessert: Berry Crumb Cake ..*page 159*

21-DAY MEAL PLAN

Day 7:
Breakfast: Apple-Banana Smoothie ..*page 40*
Snacks: Whole-Wheat–Chocolate Chip Cookies ..*page 9*
Lunch: Roasted Vegetable and White Bean Salad ..*page 81*
Snacks: Zucchini Balls With Capers And Bacon ..*page 18*
Dinner: Baked Tomato Basil Fish ..*page 119*
Dessert: Peanut Butter Oatmeal Chocolate Chip Cookies ..*page 161*

Day 8:
Breakfast: Turmeric Latte ..*page 41*
Snacks: Good-For-You Chocolate Chip Cookies ..*page 10*
Lunch: Pumpkin Seed Pesto Chicken and Arugula Sandwich ..*page 83*
Snacks: Sweet Coconut Cassava ..*page 26*
Dinner: Flavorful Grilled Shrimp ..*page 120*
Dessert: Granola Bars ..*page 163*

Day 9:
Breakfast: Herb Scrambled Egg with Asparagus ..*page 42*
Snacks: Oatmeal Sunflower Bread ..*page 11*
Lunch: Hummus Vegetable Sandwich ..*page 85*
Snacks: Tofu With Salted Caramel Pearls ..*page 27*
Dinner: Chicken Kababs ..*page 121*
Dessert: Lime Cake ..*page 165*

21-DAY MEAL PLAN

Day 10:
Breakfast: Sausage and Sauerkraut ..*page 44*
Snacks: Southwest Stuffed Avocado Bowls ..*page 12*
Lunch: Green Goddess Cucumber Tea Sandwiches ..*page 87*
Snacks: Homemade Hummus ..*page 28*
Dinner: Baked Chicken Wings ..*page 123*
Dessert: Larabar Snack Bar ..*page 169*

Day 11:
Breakfast: Banana, Flax and Turmeric Oats ..*page 45*
Snacks: Flaxseed Yogurt ..*page 14*
Lunch: Shrimp with Beans ..*page 89*
Snacks: Corn Coconut Pudding ..*page 30*
Dinner: Stuffed Sweet Potato With Hummus Dressing ..*page 137*
Dessert: Lemon Cheesecake Recipe (Limoncello Cake!) ..*page 173*

Day 12:
Breakfast: Sweet Miso Porridge ..*page 46*
Snacks: Raw Lemon Pie Bars ..*page 15*
Lunch: Broccoli Fritters ..*page 90*
Snacks: Berry Jam With Chia Seeds ..*page 31*
Dinner: Sweet Savory Hummus Plate ..*page 138*
Dessert: Hummus with Tahini and Turmeric ..*page 177*

21-DAY MEAL PLAN

Day 13:
Breakfast: Fruity Ginger Juice *..page 47*
Snacks: Trail-Mix Energy Bars *..page 16*
Lunch: Roasted Broccoli *..page 91*
Snacks: Apple Risotto *..page 32*
Dinner: Sweet Potato Black Bean Chili For Two *..page 139*
Dessert: Pineapple Orange Creamsicle *..page 178*

Day 14:
Breakfast: Pear & Celery Juice *..page 48*
Snacks: Zucchini Balls With Capers And Bacon *..page 18*
Lunch: Roasted Maple Carrots *..page 92*
Snacks: Tangy Tomato Soup *..page 2*
Dinner: Tomato Artichoke Gnocchi *..page 141*
Dessert: Easy Peach Cobbler Recipe with Bisquick *..page 179*

Day 15:
Breakfast: Apple & Cucumber Juice *..page 49*
Snacks: Sweet Orange And Lemon Barley Risotto *..page 20*
Lunch: Sweet & Tangy Green Beans *..page 93*
Snacks: Oat And Wheat Cookies *..page 3*
Dinner: Vegan Buddha Bowl *..page 143*
Dessert: Healthy 5-minute Strawberry Pineapple Sherbet *..page 181*

21-DAY MEAL PLAN

Day 16:
Breakfast: Kiwi, Apple & Cucumber Juice ..*page 50*
Snacks: Homemade Applesauce ..*page 21*
Lunch: Sautéed Carrots and Beans ..*page 94*
Snacks: Maple Oatmeal Bread ..*page 5*
Dinner: Vegan Cauliflower Fried Rice ..*page 145*
Dessert: Best Coconut Milk Ice Cream (Dairy-free!) ..*page 182*

Day 17:
Breakfast: Broccoli, Apple & Orange Juice ..*page 51*
Snacks: Homemade Beet Hummus ..*page 23*
Lunch: Antipasto on a Stick ..*page 95*
Snacks: German Dark Bread ..*page 6*
Dinner: Oatmeal Bread To Live For ..*page 147*
Dessert: Lemon Crinkle Cookies Recipe ..*page 184*

Day 18:
Breakfast: Orange & Kale Juice ..*page 52*
Snacks: Coconut Pudding With Tropical Fruit ..*page 25*
Lunch: Crab and Miso Soup ..*page 96*
Snacks: Onion And Garlic Wheat Bread ..*page 7*
Dinner: Vermicelli Puttanesca ..*page 148*
Dessert: The Best No-Bake Chocolate Lasagna ..*page 186*

21-DAY MEAL PLAN

Day 19:
Breakfast: Pear & Fennel Juice ..*page 53*
Snacks: Sweet Coconut Cassava ..*page 26*
Lunch: Mexican Lime Chicken ..*page 97*
Snacks: White Chocolate-Cranberry Cookies ..*page 8*
Dinner: Spinach And Artichoke Dip Pasta ..*page 149*
Dessert: Easiest Healthy Watermelon Smoothie Recipe ..*page 188*

Day 20:
Breakfast: Apple, Orange & Swiss Chard Juice ..*page 54*
Snacks: Tofu With Salted Caramel Pearls ..*page 27*
Lunch: Pad Thai Noodles ..*page 98*
Snacks: Whole-Wheat–Chocolate Chip Cookies ..*page 9*
Dinner: Grilled Eggplant ..*page 150*
Dessert: Baked Peanut Butter Protein Bars ..*page 164*

Day 21:
Breakfast: Carrot, Beet & Apple Juice ..*page 55*
Snacks: Homemade Hummus ..*page 28*
Lunch: Parmesan Coated Wings ..*page 99*
Snacks: Good-For-You Chocolate Chip Cookies ..*page 10*
Dinner: Tex-Mex Bean Tostadas ..*page 152*
Dessert: Banana Oatmeal Chocolate Chip Cookies (Healthy!) ..*page 167*

Conclusion

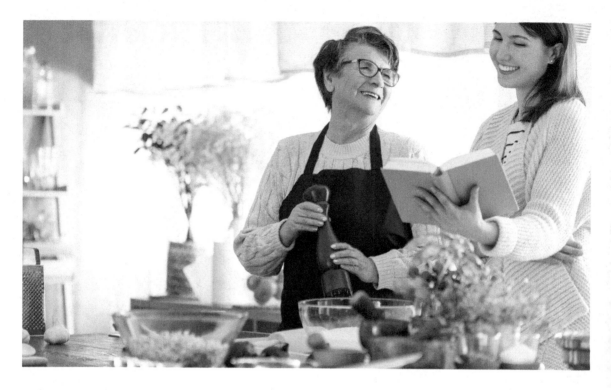

Taking a well good care of your gut is one of the major responsibilities that you need to take care of. One of the easiest ways to do so is through knowing what to eat and what not to eat!

A gut-healthy diet rich in fiber, fruits and vegetables is one of the most important ways to ensure optimal digestive health. That's because the lining of your gut wall also known as your gut microbiome is home to an army of good bacteria that help break down food and feed on certain types of food that you can't digest yourself.

This army (which includes both probiotics, which are bacteria that promote bacterial health, and prebiotics, which are fibers that promote bacterial growth) feeds on everything you put into your mouth. And when people don't eat healthy diets high in fiber, they often have fewer good bacteria supporting their gut activity—and they're more likely to get sick.

And contrary to what you might think, healthy gut bacteria are not a recent discovery. Back in the 1960s and 1970s, scientists found that people with ulcerative colitis or Crohn's disease had less good bacteria in their guts than people without those conditions. In fact, they found that the number of good microbes could predict ulcerative colitis or Crohn's disease.

More recently, though, scientists found that eating lots of fiber — especially non-starchy plant foods like fruits and vegetables — helped reshape the colonies of bacteria in your gut.

In some cases, people who ate more plant-based foods developed larger and more diverse colonies of bacteria in their guts; in others, the bacteria stayed the same but their activity increased.

More good news: Plant-based diets spread good bacteria throughout your body. Studies show that eating a diet rich in vitamins C, A and E promotes a healthier microbiome — so don't skip on fruits and vegetables just because you know you can't digest them.

There are times also when you have to deal with certain issues in your gut like bloating and constipation. You should remember that the best way to treat these issues or treat your gut is through eating the right foods!

By doing so, you can keep your digestive system going strong. the following are some of the tips on how you can fight bloating and constipation:

Bloating: To decrease bloating, eat a well-balanced diet, avoid red meat (often causes bloating), drink more water, exercise regularly and eat more high fiber vegetables.

Constipation: To decrease constipation, drink more water, eat more high fiber vegetables, and also take a B-complex vitamin.

Other helpful tips:

If your diet lacks fiber then you can start supplementing with fiber supplements. Fiber can come from different sources such as fresh fruit, vegetables and grains. A good fiber supplement that has been proven to work is called Benefiber. It comes in either chewable tablets or a powder that you mix with milk or juice. To get the best results from this, it is recommended that you take this supplement at least one hour before eating, and drink plenty of water.

Vitamin D is aalso a very important vitamin for those who want to maintain their gut health. Vitamin D is involved in the regulation of calcium and phosphorus absorption in the gut. Dietary sources include fish liver oils, eggs and fortified margarine.

Its deficiency can lead to decreased bone mineralization and increased fracture risk in postmenopausal women. Vitamin D has also been observe to have an effect on calcium metabolism in the intestines and may play a role in regulating colon cancer risk.

Iron is essential for maintaining gut health. Iron deficiency can lead to constipation, which is obviously not ideal. But here's the thing: it's almost impossible to get enough iron from your diet alone! You'd have to eat red meat every day, and even then you probably won't get enough. Consuming too much iron can also be harmful. In fact, having too much iron in your body can cause hemochromatosis, a disease that causes your body to absorb excess iron from food.

Eat a diet high in fiber. This will help to keep your digestion regular, which will prevent the colon from becoming dry, and this will prevent constipation. If you do suffer from constipation then add psyllium husks to your diet, as this can be a very effective treatment for constipation.

About
The Author

ABOUT ALLISON TUXBURY

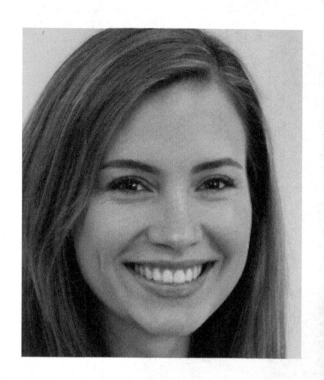

Allison Tuxbury is a professional photographer, digital graphic designer, and lover of food.

She suffered from chronic health conditions and autoimmune symptoms for nearly two decades before finding solutions in meditation, alternative medicines, energy therapy, breathwork, and nutritional meals that fuel the body.

She writes because she loves to share what she's learned with the world, and because it's fun to come up with new meals.

She hopes that through her books others who also suffer from ailments will find relief and recovery as well. She currently lives in Texas with her three children and husband.

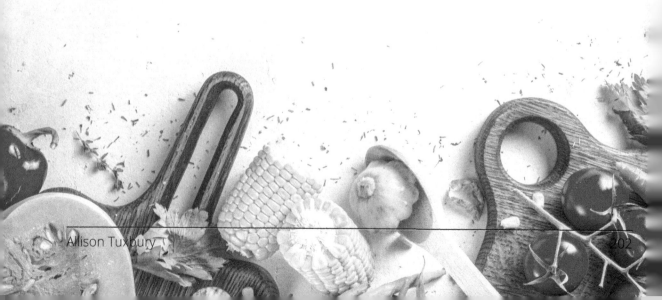

INDEX

A

- Aloe-Mint Smoothie..35
- Antipasto on a Stick..95
- Apple & Cucumber Juice..49
- Apple & Spinach Smoothie..69
- Apple Oat Smoothie..60
- Apple Risotto..32
- Apple, Orange & Swiss Chard Juice..54
- Apple, Pear & Carrot Juice..56
- Apple, Pear & Orange Juice..57
- Apple-Banana Smoothie..40

B

- Baked Chicken Wings..123
- Baked Peanut Butter Protein Bars..164
- Baked Salmon..122
- Baked Tomato Basil Fish..119
- Banana Oatmeal Chocolate Chip Cookies (Healthy!)..167
- Banana, Flax and Turmeric Oats..45
- Berry Crumb Cake..159
- Berry Flax Smoothie..38
- Berry Jam With Chia Seeds..31
- Best Coconut Milk Ice Cream (Dairy-free!)..182
- Blackberry Smoothie..62
- Blueberry & Avocado Smoothie..63
- Boiled Peanuts..22
- Bowl With Cashew Tahini Sauce..125
- Bread Pudding with Blueberries..157
- Broccoli Fritters..90
- Broccoli, Apple & Orange Juice..51

C

- Carrot and Beet Coleslaw..79
- Carrot, Beet & Apple Juice..55

- Cheeseburger Macaroni..112
- Cheesy Chicken Fritters..106
- Chicken Alfredo Pasta Bake..109
- Chicken Kababs..121
- Chocolate Butter Honey Covered Bananas..176
- Chocolate English Custard Recipes..158
- Chocolate Peanut Cookies..4
- Cinnamon Berry Smoothie..36
- Coconut Pudding With Tropical Fruit..25
- Corn Coconut Pudding..30
- Crab and Miso Soup..96
- Crispy Falafel..107
- Cucumber & Celery Smoothie..70

D

- Dark Chocolate Gelato..156
- Dark Chocolate with Pomegranate Seeds..175
- Date & Almond Smoothie..64
- Delicious Taco Chicken..117
- Deviled Egg Salad..78
- Dijon Chicken Thighs..116

E

- Easiest Healthy Watermelon Smoothie Recipe..188
- Easy Broiled Fish Fillet..118
- Easy No-Bake Key Lime Pie Recipe..171
- Easy Peach Cobbler Recipe with Bisquick..179

INDEX

F
- Flavorful Grilled Shrimp..120
- Flaxseed Yogurt..14
- Fruity Ginger Juice..47

G
- German Dark Bread..6
- Good-For-You Chocolate Chip Cookies..10
- Granola Bars..163
- Green Goddess Cucumber Tea Sandwiches..87
- Grilled Eggplant..150
- Gut-Healing Smoothie..34

H
- Healthy 5-minute strawberry pineapple sherbet..181
- Hearty Winter Salad with Forbidden Rice..80
- Herb Scrambled Egg with Asparagus..42
- Homemade Applesauce..21
- Homemade Beet Hummus..23
- Homemade Hummus..28
- Hummus Vegetable Sandwich..85
- Hummus with Tahini and Turmeric..177

K
- Kiwi & Oat Smoothie..68
- Kiwi, Apple & Cucumber Juice..50
- Kiwi, Apple & Grapes Juice..58
- Kulfi Indian Ice Cream..170

L
- Larabar Snack Bar..169
- Lemon Cheesecake Recipe (Limoncello Cake!)..173
- Lemon Chicken..115
- Lemon Crinkle Cookies Recipe..184
- Lime Cake..165

M
- Mango, Orange & Cucumber Smoothie..66
- Maple Oatmeal Bread..5
- Mexican Lime Chicken..97
- Millet Chocolate Pudding..154
- Minestrone..104
- Mushroom & Beef Bone Broth..72

O
- Oat And Wheat Cookies..3
- Oatmeal Bread To Live For..147
- Oatmeal Sunflower Bread..11
- Onion And Garlic Wheat Bread..7
- Orange & Kale Juice..52

P
- Pad Thai Noodles..98
- Parmesan Coated Wings..99
- Peach & Oat Smoothie..59
- Peanut Butter Oatmeal Chocolate Chip Cookies..161
- Pear & Almond Smoothie..65
- Pear & Celery Juice..48
- Pear & Fennel Juice..53
- Pina Colada Bites..100
- Pineapple Orange Creamsicle..178

INDEX

- Pumpkin Seed Pesto Chicken and Arugula Sandwich..83

R

- Raspberry Oat Smoothie..67
- Raw Lemon Pie Bars..15
- Rice Bean Freezer Burritos..127
- Roasted Broccoli..91
- Roasted Maple Carrots..92
- Roasted Vegetable and White Bean Salad..81
- Roasted Veggie Hummus Pita Pockets..129

S

- Salmon Skewers..114
- Sausage and Sauerkraut..44
- Sausage Peppers Baked Ziti..130
- Sauteed Butternut Squash..132
- Sautéed Carrots and Beans..94
- Savory Chicken and Rice Muffins..101
- Shiitake-Miso Cod Soup..74
- Shrimp with Beans..89
- Southwest Stuffed Avocado Bowls..12
- Spiced Sweet Potato Wedges..133
- Spicy Lemon Chicken..124
- Spinach and Aloe Smoothie..37
- Spinach And Artichoke Dip Pasta..149
- Stetson Chopped Salad..135
- Strawberry Healthy Gut Smoothie..39
- Strawberry Oat Smoothie..61
- Stuffed Sweet Potato With Hummus Dressing..137
- Sweet & Tangy Green Beans..93
- Sweet Coconut Cassava..26
- Sweet Miso Porridge..46
- Sweet Orange And Lemon Barley Risotto..20
- Sweet Potato Black Bean Chili For Two..139
- Sweet Savory Hummus Plate..138

T

- Tangy Tomato Soup..2
- Tex-Mex Bean Tostadas..152
- The Best No-bake Chocolate Lasagna..186
- Tofu With Salted Caramel Pearls..27
- Tomato Artichoke Gnocchi..141
- Trail-Mix Energy Bars..16
- Tuesday Tacos..120
- Turkey Burgers with Spinach and Feta..103
- Turmeric Latte..41

V

- Vanilla Maple Chia Pudding..154
- Vegan Buddha Bowl..143
- Vegan Cauliflower Fried Rice..145
- Vegetable-Coconut Curry Soup..76
- Vermicelli Puttanesca..148

W

- White Chocolate-Cranberry Cookies..8
- Whole-Wheat–Chocolate Chip Cookies..9

Z

- Zucchini Balls With Capers And Bacon..18

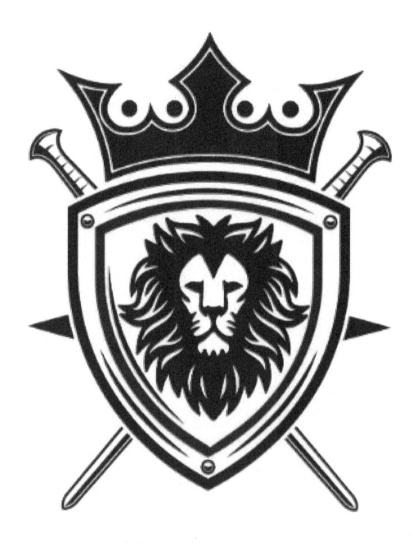

Made in the USA
Las Vegas, NV
03 February 2023

66851151R00129